Opportunities for and barriers to good nutritional health in minority ethnic groups

Foreword

This report is one of a series of linked literature reviews, commissioned by the Department of Health, as part of its commitment to protect, promote and improve the nutritional health of the nation. The aim of the series as a whole is to bring together current knowledge about cultural, behavioural, material and societal opportunities for, and barriers to, good nutritional health, so as to inform the development and implementation of interventions which are intended to encourage healthy eating in particular target groups.

This review is concerned with factors that promote healthy eating among minority ethnic groups living in Great Britain. In view of the shortage of nutrient intake studies in these groups, it focuses upon three minority ethnic groups, which are also the largest and most reported groups in which there is evidence of nutrition-related conditions: South Asians, African-Caribbeans and Irish. Other target groups which are covered in this series are:
- women of childbearing age and those who are pregnant
- infants up to one year, and from one to five
- elderly people.

There is, of course, some common ground between these reviews. For example, the present review covers the entire life cycle of the three ethnic groups under study. It therefore overlaps, to some extent, with the material covered in the other reviews of pregnant women, women of childbearing age, infants, children up to five years and elderly people. No attempt has been made to avoid overlaps and, to that extent, each of the reviews can be considered to be free-standing.

All the reviewers in this series were charged with offering pointers to new ways of formulating and delivering interventions to improve the nutritional health of target groups. Within this overall brief, they were each given the following tasks, in relation to their particular target group:
- to inform policymakers and others of what is already known about opportunities for, and barriers to, good nutritional health
- to offer suggestions on possible interventions which might be expected to overcome identified barriers or take advantage of identified opportunities, which could then be tested in further research
- to inform the design of future dietary intervention strategies to improve their effectiveness

- to identify needs for further research and appropriate research questions.

In parallel with this series of reviews of opportunities for, and barriers to, healthy eating, the Department of Health also commissioned a second set of literature reviews which focus upon the effectiveness of interventions to promote healthier eating, in the same target groups. This parallel set of reviews, commissioned through the Health Education Authority in their series, Health promotion effectiveness reviews, focuses explicitly upon the methods, outcomes and effectiveness of existing interventions. Our own series deals with interventions only in so far as they throw light upon the barriers to, or opportunities for, dietary change which are our primary focus. As a result, the two sets of reviews are complementary to one another. All of these reviews are concerned with factors which influence the dietary behaviours of the healthy population, rather than with the treatment or care of those who are ill. The focus is upon factors which either facilitate or obstruct healthy eating among members of each target group. All the reviewers have taken as their starting point the current best advice on diet and nutrition for the whole population, which is embodied in COMA reports (Department of Health and Social Security, 1988; Department of Health, 1991; 1992a; 1994a; 1994b; 1997). They have been concerned to identify ways in which the nutrition targets set out in the *Health of the Nation* White Paper (Department of Health, 1992b) may be met. These targets are summarised in Figure 1.

Saturated fat
To reduce the average percentage of food energy derived by the population from saturated fatty acids by at least 35% by 2005 (from 17% in 1990 to no more than 11%).

Total fat
To reduce the average percentage of food energy derived by the population from total fat by at least 12% by 2005 (from about 40% in 1990 to no more than 35%).

Fig. 1. Relevant Health of the Nation targets (Department of Health, 1992b)

For the purposes of these reviews, 'healthy eating' is defined as eating behaviours which are compatible with achieving the dietary reference values (Department of Health, 1991), which meet these Health of the Nation targets (Department of Health, 1992b). Such 'healthy eating' involves eating the foods from the five food groups in the proportions set out in *The balance of good health* (Health Education Authority, 1995) and summarised in Figure 2.

- Eating lots of *bread, other cereals and potatoes* and choosing wholemeal, wholegrain or high fibre versions where possible. Avoiding, where possible, fried versions, adding too much fat or rich sauces and dressings.

- Eating lots of *fruit and vegetables* and choosing a wide variety. Avoiding, where possible, adding fat or rich sauces to vegetables and sugar to fruit.

- Eating or drinking moderate amounts of *milk and dairy foods* and choosing lower fat versions where possible.

- Eating moderate amounts of *meat, fish and alternatives* and choosing lower fat versions where possible.

- Eating foods containing *fat* sparingly, choosing *low fat alternatives* and eating *foods containing sugar* not too often.

Fig. 2. **Means by which 'healthy eating' may be achieved**

Food group	Foods	Recommended behaviour for healthy eating
Bread, other cereals and potatoes	Bread and rolls	Eat lots and choose wholemeal, wholegrain, brown or high fibre versions where possible. Avoid adding too much butter, margarine or low fat spread.
	Breakfast cereals	Eat lots and choose high fibre types where possible.
	Pasta, rice and other grains	Eat lots, try brown where possible and avoid adding rich sauces and dressings.
	Potatoes	Eat lots, with the skin on if possible and avoid having them fried too often or served with fat spread.
Fruit and vegetables	Fruit	Eat lots, include a variety and avoid adding sugar or syrupy dressings.
	Vegetables	Eat lots, include a variety and avoid adding butter, margarine, fat spread or rich sauces.
	Salad vegetables	Eat lots, include a variety and avoid mayonnaise and oily dressings where possible.
Milk and dairy products	Milk	Drink moderate amounts and choose semi-skimmed or skimmed where possible.
	Cheese	Eat moderate amounts and choose lower fat cheeses such as Edam, half-fat Cheddar or Camembert.
	Yoghurt and fromage frais	Eat moderate amounts and choose low fat (0.1%) rather than whole milk products.
Meat, fish and alternatives	Meat (includes carcass meat and meat products)	Eat moderate amounts of lean meat with the fat cut off, and cook without added fat and limit the amount and frequency of eating high fat meat products such as pies and pasties.
	Poultry	Eat moderate amounts, without the skin and cook without added fat.
	Fish	Eat moderate amounts, without added fat or batter and eat oily fish twice weekly.
	Eggs	Eat moderate amounts and avoid frying or adding fat where possible.
	Beans	Eat moderate amounts as a naturally low fat alternative to meat.
Foods containing fat Foods containing sugar	Spreading fats: butter, margarine, reduced fat spread	Can be eaten daily, but in very small amounts. Choose low fat alternatives.
	Cooking oils	Can be eaten daily, but in small amounts.
	Mayonnaise and oil-based salad dressings	Can be used daily but in very small amounts. Choose low fat alternatives.
	Cakes, biscuits, pastries, confectionery, crisps, cream, soft drinks	Limit amount and frequency of eating and choose lower fat alternatives. If foods and drinks contain sugar, limit to mealtimes.

Fig. 3. **Healthy eating behaviours**

Based on guidance provided by the Health Education Authority, Department of Health and MAFF in: *The balance of good health: information for educators and communicators* (Health Education Authority, 1995).

The eating behaviours which are compatible with healthy eating include, but are not restricted to those listed in Figure 3. Nutritional issues which are specific to the minority ethnic groups considered here are discussed in Chapters 2, 3 and 4 under 'Culture and food choice'.

Elizabeth Murphy
Series Co-ordinator and Editor
School of Social Studies
University of Nottingham

References

Department of Health and Social Security (1988). *Present day practice in infant feeding: third report*. Report on Health and Social Subjects No. 32. London: HMSO.

Department of Health (1991). *Dietary reference values for food energy and nutrients for the United Kingdom*. Report of the Panel on Dietary Reference Values of the Committee on Medical Aspects of Food Policy. Report on Health and Social Subjects No. 41. London: HMSO.

Department of Health (1992a). *The nutrition of elderly people*. Report of the Working Group of the Committee on Medical Aspects of Food Policy. Report on Health and Social Subjects No. 43. London: HMSO.

Department of Health (1992b). *The health of the nation: a strategy for health in England*. London: HMSO.

Department of Health (1994a). *Weaning and the weaning diet*. Report of the Working Group on the Weaning Diet of the Committee on Medical Aspects of Food Policy. Report on Health and Social Subjects No. 45. London: HMSO.

Department of Health (1994b). *Nutritional aspects of cardiovascular disease*. Report of the Cardiovascular Review Group Committee on Medical Aspects of Food Policy. Report on Health and Social Subjects No. 46. London: HMSO.

Department of Health (1997). *Nutritional aspects of the development of cancer*. Report of the Cancer Review Group of the Committee of Medical Aspects of Food and Nutrition Policy. Report on Health and Social Subjects No. 48. London: HMSO.

Health Education Authority (1995). *The balance of good health: information for educators and communicators*. London: Health Education Authority.

Acknowledgements

We thank the staff of the document delivery service at the University of Glasgow Library for processing inter-library loans. We are grateful to Janie Ferguson and Felicity Grainger, Glasgow University Library, for database searches and to Mary Robins at the MRC Medical Sociology Unit for obtaining references from a range of sources. Sharon Friel, National Nutrition Surveillance Centre, University College Galway and John Eade, Department of Sociology and Social Policy, Roehampton Institute, London, kindly provided us with material. Leena Seevak and Paul McKeigue, of the Department of Epidemiology and Population Sciences, London School of Hygiene and Tropical Medicine, gave details of their intervention studies in South Asians. Sumithra Muthayya, Nutrition Research Centre, St John's Medical College, Bangalore and Prakesh Shetty, London School of Hygiene and Tropical Medicine generously provided us with details of breast-feeding rates from their unpublished study in Bangalore, India.

We thank Liz Dowler, Centre for Human Nutrition, London School of Hygiene and Tropical Medicine, and Margot Barker, Centre for Human Nutrition, University of Sheffield for information on current research in the Irish community in Britain. We are very grateful to Annie Anderson, School of Management and Consumer Studies, University of Dundee for reading sections of the text, and for providing clarification of technical issues, and we thank Sally Macintyre, MRC Medical Sociology Unit, Glasgow for reading the first draft.

This work received funding from the Department of Health; the views expressed in this publication are those of the authors and not necessarily those of the Department of Health.

1. Background

Minority ethnic groups were identified in the Department of Health's document *R & D priorities in nutrition* as a priority area requiring the identification of dietary intakes and nutrition problems.

Our focus is ethnic minorities in Great Britain, and the world literature is considered only where relevant.

The nutrition and diet of ethnic minorities in Great Britain are covered very unevenly in the research literature. Clues therefore have to be sought in any excess of nutrition-related conditions. On this basis the groups considered here are South Asians (problems of heart disease, central obesity, vitamin D and iron deficiency and low birthweight), African-Caribbeans (obesity and stroke), and Irish (generalised high mortality and short stature suggesting the possibility of some vulnerability factor associated with low income, possibly nutritional). Of these groups, the literature on South Asians is by far the biggest.

2. South Asians

Data on dietary intakes of South Asian adults generally are few because of the concentration in the past on specific groups perceived to be particularly at risk of nutritional deficiencies. This bias has determined the material available to the present review ('Nutritional issues' in Section 1).

The literature concentrates on issues of diet in pregnancy, birthweight, iron and vitamin D deficiency, rickets/osteomalacia and tuberculosis, with attention being paid more recently to coronary heart disease (CHD), diabetes and obesity ('Nutritional issues' in Section 1).

The presence of diet-related conditions in South Asian groups is frequently viewed as a consequence of cultural differences which are interpreted as deficiencies, and socioeconomic disadvantage is seldom considered. This review has pointed to barriers to sound nutritional health in ethnic minorities presented by low income ('Access' in Section 2, and Section 3 'Looking to the future').

In other parts of the literature the concern is for access to culturally appropriate food on the assumption that it is healthy. While this should not always be assumed, there is enough truth in the assumption for this literature to indicate useful opportunities for sound nutritional health ('Access' in Section 2).

Following on from this, there is a range of evidence for the failure to provide culturally appropriate foods in institutional settings, affecting all age groups ('Access' in Section 2).

Issues of information are a recurring theme in the literature; both content and communication of information present potential barriers to good nutritional health ('Access' in Section 2).

The review has highlighted the need for health professionals and other service providers to have a sound knowledge of South Asian lifestyles in order to make more appropriate the information and services which they provide (Section 2).

There are differences in dietary practices between South Asian sub-groups which may be important for the promotion of sound nutritional health ('Culture and food choice' in Section 2). Conditions related to vegetarianism, and to infant feeding, have received considerable attention, with conflicting conclusions.

Interventions aimed at reducing CHD, obesity, rickets/osteomalacia and infant health are described. The high rates of CHD in South Asians were more recently recognised so relevant interventions and their evaluation are currently very limited. Interventions aimed at reducing vitamin D deficiency and rickets/osteomalacia have had variable success, and the best preventive steps have yet to be decided. The Asian Mother and Baby Campaign overcame some barriers identified in 'Access' and 'Culture and food choice' but not others ('Intervention with South Asians' in Section 2).

Practical suggestions for potential interventions, the enhancement of future dietary intervention strategies and research priorities are made in the areas of general health, CHD and control of obesity, conditions related to vegetarianism, and infant feeding and infant health (Section 4).

3. African-Caribbeans
Very little nutrition research has been carried out in the British African-Caribbean population in the last 35 years. To date, the largest study has been undertaken in Manchester on some 250 subjects ('Nutritional issues' in Section 1).

This study and some smaller, less quantitative ones have shown African-Caribbean dietary intakes to be lower in fat and higher in carbohydrate than the diets of the white population, but have also revealed high rates of obesity ('Nutritional issues' in Section 1).

The general message is thus potentially very positive – that dietary quality is excellent (being already better than national COMA recommendations) but quantity needs to be either reduced or balanced by greater physical activity ('Nutritional issues' in Section 1).

Positive results are strongest among those who eat traditional foods ('Culture and food choice' in Section 2); but traditional foods are expensive because imported, and African-Caribbeans are more socioeconomically disadvantaged than whites ('Access' in Section 2).

Further work needs to assess nutritional intakes of this population, both elsewhere in the UK and among people of Eastern Caribbean, as distinct from mainly Jamaican, origin (Section 4).

Work is also required to examine energy balance (i.e. intake and expenditure) in relation to development of health problems, including diabetes, high blood pressure and resulting cardiovascular disease, and effective intervention methods for restraining weight gain and later obesity and its consequences (Section 4).

These biomedical issues need to be examined in a culturally appropriate context, bearing in mind that positive attitudes to greater weight (which are not themselves well documented) may be prevalent ('Culture and food choice' in Section 2).

4. The Irish

Almost nothing in the literature addresses the diet and nutrition of the Irish in Britain, a serious deficit in the face of increasing evidence of health disadvantage in a wide range of conditions, including CHD and cancer, which persists among the British-born. In the past this has not usually been explicable by high mortality in Ireland ('Nutritional issues' in Section 1).

Reduced stature of Catholics of Irish descent in Scotland has been reported, which is likely to be a legacy of deprivation, including inadequate nutrition ('Nutritional issues' in Section 1).

Food consumption patterns and nutrient intakes of the Irish Republic and Northern Ireland are compared with those in Britain, and potential nutritional influences on CHD, obesity and cancers are examined ('Nutritional issues' in Section 1).

Poverty and solitary living may be barriers to nutritional health for the elderly Irish (especially male) in Britain; subject to return migration, the percentage of Irish of pensionable age is set to increase markedly in the coming decades ('Access' in Section 2, and Section 3).

Because of the shortage of British data, social class and food choice in Ireland are considered to estimate possible responses of Irish migrants, who are socioeconomically disadvantaged in Britain (Section 1 and 'Access' in Section 2).

High intakes of dietary fat and low intakes of fibre have previously been linked to CHD, cancers and obesity, and Irish attitudes to these elements vary by social class, gender and age (Section 2).

Reports suggest that the Irish population does not perceive CHD to be a major health problem in Ireland, nor appreciate that preventive measures can be taken ('Culture and food choice' in Section 2).

Some standard interventions concerned with growth monitoring, CHD and bowel cancer may be directed towards people of Irish descent in Britain ('Practical suggestions' in Section 4).

There is considerable scope for the collection of basic nutritional data, for analysis of nutrition-related data which may help to explain excess mortality among the Irish in Britain, and for collection of other, descriptive data on potential areas for intervention ('Research priorities' in Section 4).

1. Background

Definition of terms

'South Asian' is a collective term used to describe those born in or with a line of descent from India, Pakistan or Bangladesh. As a description it is preferable to 'Asian' since it differentiates other Asian nationalities such as the Chinese; however, it is an artificial category which obscures not only the cultural and religious differences which exist between the national and sub-national groups, but also their widely-differing social and economic circumstances and demographic patterns. All these variables impinge upon dietary practices, which themselves vary between groups.

The terms 'African-Caribbean' (AfC) (previously Afro-Caribbean) and 'Black Caribbean' refer to people who are of Caribbean origin but of (west) African descent. Most people over 45 years migrated as young people. This review does not include people who have migrated directly from west Africa whose culture and nutrition is quite separate from African-Caribbeans, although brief reference is made to the two other Black groups in Great Britain categorised in the 1991 Census as 'Black – African' and 'Black – Other'. African-American refers to people in the United States who are of African descent, generally also descendants of people who survived slavery. Literature on African-Americans has been excluded from this review except in the section on interventions, as American food and nutrient intake and factors affecting these are quite different to those in Britain.

The term 'Black' has been used in the past for political reasons as a description of appearance which constantly gives rise to discrimination in 'White' (European) populations and also as a way of identifying a culture (Azuonye, 1996). Throughout this review the term has only been used when describing studies that have identified the subjects reported in no other way than 'Black'.

Comparisons between these minority ethnic groups and others introduces the vexed question of the name by which the latter should be described. 'White' is the term commonly resorted to but is undesirable since it implies that ethnicity is synonymous with race. 'Caucasian', 'white Caucasian' and 'European' are also in general use. We have employed the term 'ethnic majority', but have retained the descriptions used by the authors of the studies we cite.

The use of the term 'white' also obscures important ethnic differences within the 'white' group. As a 'white' minority, the Irish have received little attention during the postwar period, though this was far from being the case during the nineteenth century. In line with the other definitions given above, the term Irish is used to include those born in or with a line of descent from Ireland. Religious divisions between Catholic and Protestant Irish, and political divisions between the Republic and Northern Ireland, make for heterogeneity among Irish groups. At the same time the extent to which these different religious and ethnic identities have been diluted by intermarriage with the general British population remains unclear. These aspects are discussed in more detail in Section 1 of Chapter 4.

Scope: ethnic minorities in Great Britain

The focus of this review is ethnic minorities in Great Britain, and the world literature is considered only where relevant. Identifying ethnic minorities in Britain is difficult because of the classification system used by the Census. The full ethnic group classification employed in the 1991 Census uses 35 categories which are generally condensed into a 10-category classification in most statistical output (Appendix B), the full classification being used in a single table of Census statistics (Aspinall, 1996). Numerically smaller groups and those newest to Great Britain are not differentiated. For example, the 'Other – Asian' category contains within it 'Other Asian', into which such groups as Japanese, Korean, Malays and Filipinos are amalgamated. Nor are refugee groups such as Vietnamese, Somalis, Sri Lankans and Kurds differentiated; the Vietnamese community has existed in Britain for many years but the data are lacking which could illuminate its circumstances and aid in the design and monitoring of policies to improve its situation and that of the other refugee groups (Owen, 1996).

Identification of ethnic groups is complicated further by the fact that the Census (like numerous other bodies) does not currently allow for the identification of ethnic groups among the majority white population. Thus any who identify themselves as 'Irish', 'Greek', 'Turkish' or 'Other European' are lost in the process of condensation into the 'white' category (see Appendix B). At the 1991 Census there were in excess of one and a half million people living in Britain who were born in the European Union, the remainder of Europe and the Old Commonwealth and USA (Compton, 1996). Although being born in these regions obviously does not directly equate with being 'white', the figure provides an indication of the potential size of 'hidden' ethnic minorities in Great Britain.

Currently the range of ethnic minorities in Great Britain can only be determined from place of birth statistics, but it is known that these do not necessarily indicate national origin and they are not good estimators of the size of ethnic groups (Compton, 1996). Thus we have an imperfect picture of the ethnic composition of Great Britain, but in pointing out the shortcomings of the Census we should note that it is not intended to function 'as a data source for social scientists' (Compton, 1996, p. 243), and that ways of improving the ethnic group question for the 2001 Census are being explored (Aspinall, 1996).

Relevance of three main Great Britain ethnic minorities to Department of Health priorities in nutrition

The nutrition and diet of ethnic minorities in Great Britain are covered very unevenly in the research literature. Nutrient intake studies are available in only a few cases and, in their absence, clues have to be sought in any excess of nutrition-related disease, of low birthweight, of obesity, of short stature, or of high mortality across a large number of disease categories including infections. On this basis the groups considered here are South Asians (problems of heart disease, central obesity, vitamin D and iron deficiency and low birthweight), African-Caribbeans (obesity and stroke), and Irish (generalised high mortality and short stature suggesting the possibility of some vulnerability factor associated with low income, possibly nutritional). This approach is in line with the Department of Health's commissioning document's specification of 'the need to outline issues relating to the health of target groups' and to review 'current nutritional intake and dietary behaviour'. These three minorities are also rendered central because they contain groups with relatively large numbers of children and sizeable groups on low income, children and those on low income being two other priority groups in the Department of Health's *R & D priorities in nutrition*. Among these three ethnic minorities, the largest literature is on South Asians and the smallest on the Irish.

Nutritional issues in other ethnic minorities in Great Britain

In order to make a broad estimate of the volume of relevant material concerning other ethnic minorities in Great Britain, which might be buried under national titles only without reference to ethnicity or race, we selected the Black African and Chinese groups (since they are the largest ethnic groups aside from 'white', African-Caribbean and the three main South Asian groups) and searched BIDS (Social Sciences Citation Index) from 1981 to 1996 since this database was prolific in terms of South Asian references. This produced one reference, indicating a gap in published material on ethnic minorities other than the three selected here concerning issues relevant to this review.

Overview of available literature: scope and methods

Differing economic and political backgrounds and geographical contexts mean that studies of South Asians and African-Caribbeans from outside Britain could not usefully be included, but in the absence of British material the review of African-Caribbeans has made limited use of references to black Americans. In the general absence of studies of the Irish in Britain, the Irish literature was used and was traced mainly through bibliographies of studies and reports (primarily publications of the National Nutrition Surveillance Centre, University College Galway) since little appeared on the databases.

Search methods

The keywords used and databases searched are listed in Appendix C. A cut-off point of 1980 has been agreed for all reviews, although the possibility of tracing back further for any known topics for which earlier literature is relevant was also agreed. The review is confined to English-language publications. Additional examples of 'grey' literature could be assembled through informal contacts, but in the face of time constraints it was felt that the yield of information in such studies was likely to be relatively low.

Criteria for assessing the quality of the studies/minimum methodological criteria for inclusion

Because of the limited amount of literature concerned with ethnic minorities there were no minimum methodological criteria for inclusion, but details of the design of data studies are given in Appendix A to permit their evaluation by users of this document.

Procedures for extracting data from studies

A pro forma common to the three reviews was used to ensure uniform extraction and comparability of data from studies.

2. South Asians

1. South Asians in context

The 1991 Census reported a little under 1.5 million South Asians living in Great Britain, forming 2.7% of the population (Peach, 1996). We have described how the term 'South Asian' obscures important differences between national and sub-national groups and, although much of the research literature on the health of South Asians ignores these differences (Ahmad *et al.*, 1989), it is essential for assessment to be made at sub-national level wherever possible.

Indians are the largest South Asian group in Britain, numbering 840 255 at the 1991 Census, and Bangladeshis the smallest at 162 835. The Pakistani group lies between the two, numbering 476 555 (Peach, 1996). Ballard (1996) reviews the inherent difficulties of 'Bangladeshi' and 'Pakistani' as markers of ethnic identity, in the light of the recent formation of these countries; we use them without qualification as reported in the 1991 Census.

South Asian migration to Britain is not a recent process, for there has been an Indian presence since the eighteenth century at least (Robinson, 1996, p. 95). With the exception of those forced to leave East Africa on political grounds in the 1960s and 70s, more recent migration has been motivated by economic factors, with the large-scale labour migration occurring in the 1950s and 60s. Until the 1950s migrants were mainly Gujarati Indians, but from the 1950s onwards men from the Punjab (Indian and Pakistani) and Kashmir (Pakistan) came to Britain and were followed by their families in the 1960s and 70s. Migration from the Sylhet district of what is now Bangladesh is more recent, from the 1970s (Eade, Vamplew and Peach, 1996).

The following is derived from detailed analyses of the circumstances of Indians (Robinson, 1996), Pakistanis (Ballard, 1996) and Bangladeshis (Eade, Vamplew and Peach, 1996) and the overview of the South Asian population in Britain (Owen, 1994a) which have been produced since the publication of the 1991 Census Data.

Geographical distribution, economic situation and income
Geographical distribution
Indians are almost entirely resident in England (with only 0.4% of

Indians in the UK in Scotland and 0.6% in Wales) and primarily in the West and East Midlands and especially in the South East. By contrast, Pakistanis live generally in northern England (particularly West Yorkshire and the North West) and the West Midlands metropolitan counties. Bangladeshis are most geographically concentrated, especially in Greater London where more than half the British Bangladeshi population resides. Almost a quarter (23%) of Bangladeshis in Britain live in Tower Hamlets (Eade, Vamplew and Peach, 1996); not surprisingly the majority of studies of Bangladeshis have been carried out in this London borough, which inevitably limits what can be extrapolated to other Bangladeshis in Britain, who are mainly in the West Midlands metropolitan county and Greater Manchester.

Economic situation

Marked differences exist in the economic circumstances of South Asian groups in Britain, with Indians and East African Asians enjoying a better situation overall than Pakistanis and, especially, Bangladeshis.

Employment

Indian men are almost as likely as 'white' and more likely than Pakistani and Bangladeshi men to be economically active, that is either to be employed or to be actively seeking work. Considerably fewer women in all three groups are economically active, particularly Pakistani and Bangladeshi women, possibly reflecting the conventional domestic role of Muslim women. The material circumstances of the family has been shown to be an important factor in whether Muslim women work (Brah and Shaw, 1992, p. 49). Table 9 details economic activity.

South Asians generally are less likely than the ethnic majority to be in managerial positions or skilled manual jobs, but more likely to be doctors, proprietors or semi-skilled workers. Indian and Pakistani men work predominantly in engineering, distribution, transport/communications and business services; the textile and clothing industry is particularly important for Pakistanis, but they are less likely than Indians or 'whites' to work in business services or the public sector. By contrast, more than two-thirds of Bangladeshi men work in retailing and catering. Indian and Pakistani women work in similar fields to men in these minorities, but also in health and education, while Bangladeshi women tend to work in distribution, textiles/clothing and health and education (Brah and Shaw, 1992).

Self-employment is an important mode of working for South Asians (Table 9), more so than for 'whites'. Ballard (1996) notes that the term covers a wide range of work and statuses; while Bangladeshi men are most likely to be employees (probably as a consequence of their marked involvement in the catering industry), Indian men are more likely than other South Asian men to be self-employed professionals, probably 'the most prosperous area'. Pakistanis are prominent in non-professional self-employment, typically taxi driving.

The high rates of self-employment complicate analysis of South Asian social class distribution, since many self-employed are conventionally placed in Class II. However, Peach (1996, p. 16) has looked at ethnic groups in the 1991 Census in terms of proportions in the professional classes, showing a little over 11% of Indian men in Social Class I, considerably more than Pakistani (5.9%), Bangladeshi (5.2%) and white (6.7%) men. Pakistanis and Bangladeshis are also skewed towards the manual end of the distribution, despite figuring in the managerial classes (Peach, 1996), with 55% of Pakistani men and 63% of Bangladeshi men aged 16 and over in manual employment (Classes III (Manual), IV and V) (Ballard, 1996). Analysis of women in terms of social class is less useful, particularly for Pakistanis and Bangladeshis because of their low rate of economic activity, but Indians are more likely than other South Asians or white women to be in Class I (Table 10).

Unemployment

Major differences exist in the unemployment rates of men in the South Asian groups, with rates for Indians lying well below those of Pakistanis and Bangladeshis (Table 9). The unemployment rates of Bangladeshi men (30.9%) and women (34.5%) are 'massively high' (Eade, Vamplew and Peach, 1996, p. 155), despite the low percentage of women seeking work. Rates for Pakistani men (28.5%) and women (29.6%) are almost as high, but are much lower for Indians (13.4% and 12.7%). Differential rates of unemployment partly reflect educational attainment, a higher percentage of Indians and a lower percentage of Pakistanis and Bangladeshis having further and higher British education qualifications than 'white' Britons. However, unemployment rates for highly-qualified South Asians are considerably greater than for 'whites'.

Income

Recent data concerning the earnings of British ethnic minorities are limited, but figures for 1994–95 from the Office for National Statistics indicate that the considerable earnings differentials noted by Jones (1993) continue: in terms of average full-time hourly earnings, Indian men (£8.01) come closest to 'white' (£8.34), with Pakistani and Bangladeshi men earning considerably less (£6.87). Indian women's hourly pay (£5.75) is also closer to white women (£6.59), although the difference between them is greater than between Indian and 'white' men, and is even more so for Pakistani and Bangladeshi women (£4.78) (Church and Summerfield, 1996). Regional studies confirm this differential – a survey in Leicester in 1990, for example, showed that male South Asians earned approximately 80% of the 'white' wage (Jones, 1993); women's wages are not referred to.

Housing tenure

Indians and Pakistanis have very high rates of owner occupation at 82% and 77% respectively, compared to 'whites' (67%). Many fewer Bangladeshis are owner occupiers (45%), but this is partly due to their high concentration in Tower Hamlets where owner occupation has not been common. Even allowing for this, Bangladeshis are over-represented in local authority housing by about 17%. South Asians are more likely than 'whites' to experience overcrowding, non-exclusive use of bath/WC and lack of central heating. Pakistanis and Bangladeshis have the largest households of the South Asian groups, and with 8% and 19% respectively living with more than 1.5 persons per room, are more likely than Indians and 'whites' to suffer overcrowding. Pakistanis and especially Bangladeshis are much less likely to have central heating than Indians and 'whites', a fact possibly explained for Pakistanis in that their lower incomes encourage the purchase of older housing lacking this amenity.

Age and gender structure, family composition

South Asians are younger than the white ethnic majority on average. Indians (median age c.28 years) are older on average than Pakistanis (median age c.20) and Bangladeshis (median age c.17). Bangladeshis, though generally youthful, differ from other South Asians in that there are considerably more men than women in the 50–65 age group, a reflection of the later family reunification of Bangladeshis than of other South Asian groups. The highest percentage of people of pensionable age occurs for Indian females (6.6%). The number of children younger than 4 years is smaller than those aged 5–9 in all South Asian groups, indicating a slowing down in population growth. Two-fifths of all Indians are UK-born, half of all Pakistanis and a third of all Bangladeshis. Males are in the majority, except in age groups 20–24 and 25–29, although men of these ages were underestimated at the last Census (Owen, 1994a).

Table 11 details marital status and family composition. A final issue relevant to the current review is that of unsupported claims which have been made for the 'disintegration of the Asian traditional family unit' (Aslam and Healey, 1982, p. 1354), and the suggestion that the extended family in Britain is a 'myth' (e.g. Ali and Begum, 1991). These claims arise from figures which show a high frequency of nuclear South Asian households with only nine per cent of Indians, Pakistanis and Bangladeshis living in households with two or more families (Ballard, 1996). The figures have been dismissed by Ballard in his analysis of Pakistanis from the 1991 Census data, who argues that the trend is illusory and stems from the constraints imposed by British housing stock.

Nutritional issues

Data on dietary intakes of South Asian adults generally are few because, until recently, attention has been focused on specific groups perceived to be particularly at risk from nutritional deficiencies, notably:

1. *South Asian women in pregnancy* (Abraham *et al.*, 1985; Campbell-Brown *et al.*, 1985; Abraham *et al.*, 1987; Ward *et al.*, 1988; Viegas *et al.*, 1982a, 1982b; Eaton, Wharton and Wharton, 1984; Wharton, Eaton and Wharton, 1984). Reported intakes of protein, energy, iron and vitamin D have been highlighted, with many intakes at the lower end of the range considered inadequate. Biochemical evidence for vitamin D deficiency has been presented (Bashir, Macdonald and Peacock, 1981). Studies reporting intakes of these nutrients are detailed in Table 1.

2. *South Asian babies* Low birthweight has been reported compared to those of the ethnic majority (e.g. Davies *et al.*, 1982; McFadyen *et al.*, 1984). Assessments of the extent of the problem vary (Clarson *et al.*, 1982; Versi *et al.*, 1995). The causes are debated but may include maternal undernutrition (Davies *et al.*, 1982; Mason, Davies and Marshall, 1982; Versi *et al.*, 1995; Viegas *et al.*, 1982b; Wharton and Wharton, 1989). Brook and Wood (1980) have argued that vitamin D deficiency may reduce birthweight. Variations in birthweight have been reported by religion and whether migrant or British-born (McFadyen *et al.*, 1984; Dhawan, 1995; Draper, Abrams and Clarke, 1995).

3. *Young South Asian children* because of concern about iron deficiency anaemia (Harris *et al.*, 1983; Ehrhardt, 1986; Grindulis *et al.*, 1986; Warrington and Storey, 1988b; Harbottle and Duggan, 1992; Duggan *et al.*, 1991), although iron deficiency is also the principal cause of anaemia in children in the UK generally (James and Laing, 1994). Increased risk is associated with prematurity, prolonged exclusive breast-feeding, a weaning diet deficient in iron (Department of Health, 1994b), late weaning (James and Laing, 1994) and low income (Low Income Project Team, 1996). However, a study of South Asian children in Sheffield found evidence of adequate growth despite high prevalence of anaemia (Duggan *et al.*, 1991) and Moore and Worwood (1989) suggest that low levels of iron may have some connection with the low rates of sudden infant death syndrome which have been reported for South Asians (Hilder, 1994; Balarajan, Sonny and Botting, 1989). Older children may also be affected by iron deficiency anaemia (Nelson, Bakalion and Trivedi, 1994; Agha *et al.*, 1992).

4. *Young South Asian children, adolescents and adult women* because of concern about rickets, osteomalacia and vitamin D deficiency (Dunnigan *et al.*, 1962; Ford *et al.*, 1972; Robertson *et al.*, 1982; Henderson *et al.*, 1990; Harris *et al.*, 1983; Iqbal *et al.*, 1994; Solanki *et al.*, 1995). Supplementary vitamin D has been recommended for South Asian women and children (Department of Health, 1991). Rickets may also be caused by coeliac disease (Thalayasing, 1985), from which British

Punjabis in particular have been reported as being at high risk (Sher *et al.*, 1993), although actual numbers affected are very small. 'Asian rickets' is a commonly used (e.g. Ford, 1974; Robertson, 1982; Clements, 1990; Smith, 1990) but incorrect term since it implies the 'racial specificity' of the condition (Ahmad, 1989, p. 14).

5. South Asian tuberculosis sufferers TB is a disease of poverty (Mangtani *et al.*, 1995), but the increased risk of South Asians (1992 CMO Report on State of the Public Health, cited by Karmi and McKeigue, 1993) has been attributed to vegetarian diet (Finch, Millard and Maxwell, 1991; Strachan *et al.*, 1995). The process is unknown, but the impact of vitamin D deficiency upon immunocompetence was suggested (Strachan *et al.*, 1995). Religious and gender differences in risk have been noted (Ormerod *et al.*, 1991; Bakhshi, 1993). A decrease in South Asian cases has been reported in Birmingham since 1981 (Bakhshi, 1993).

Because of the earlier focus on these specific groups, information about the nutrient intakes of 'healthy' individuals is minimal. Recently, though, the growing awareness of the elevated rates of coronary heart disease (CHD) and obesity in migrant South Asians has encouraged people to undertake surveys of the working adult population. Death rates from CHD are higher in migrants from the Indian sub-continent than in the general population of the UK (Marmot, Adelstein and Bulusi, 1984; Balarajan and Bulusu, 1990; Balarajan, 1996). The high rates are common to the main South Asian groups in the UK, and also occur in South Asian migrants worldwide and in urban Indian populations, and cannot be explained by the classic risk factors of hypertension, smoking and high serum cholesterol (McKeigue, Miller and Marmot, 1989; Knight *et al.*, 1992). Analysis of seven-day weighed intake data collected from South Asian (mainly Punjabi Sikh) and European men in London concluded that no unfavourable characteristic of the South Asian diet could account for high rates of CHD (Sevak, McKeigue and Marmot, 1994), but results from other studies in Table 2 suggest a more variable picture with some high mean total percentage intakes from fat. Further, Thompson and Cruickshank (1990) report very low intakes of fatty acids normally obtained from fish oils in vegetarian Gujerati women. Changeover to Western diet in South Asian students may also be related to elevated total serum cholesterol (Potts and Simmons, 1994). However, the underlying problem signalled by high prevalence of non-insulin dependent diabetes, central obesity and CHD may be a syndrome of insulin resistance (Karmi and McKeigue, 1993; McKeigue, Shah and Marmot, 1991; Bose, 1995; Gishen, Hogh and Stock, 1995; Wardle, Wrightson and Gibson, 1996), possibly inherited (Shaukat, de Bono and Jones, 1995), though the syndrome may be more a mechanism than a cause of high rates of disease (Cruickshank, 1995; Frayn, Williams and Arner, 1996).

McKeigue and Chaturvedi (1996, p. 57) argue that obesity is 'probably the most important target variable to control' in South Asians. Criteria for ideal body weight in South Asian communities have not been defined: inter-group differences in weight-for-height have been reported (McKeigue *et al.*, 1988; McKeigue, Shah and Marmot, 1991) and may indicate differences in body frame size rather than the amount of body fat. McKeigue and Chaturvedi argue that South Asians with a BMI > 27 and waist/hip ratio greater than 1.00 (men) or 0.87 (women) should be targeted in health-care programmes. Anthropometric data from a number of studies are presented in Table 3.

McKeigue and Chaturvedi also propose a reduction in dietary fat intake as the most effective tool. They describe the COMA target of 33% of total energy intake (including alcohol) as 'probably too conservative' (p. 58) – though surveys reported in Table 2 show mean total energy intake to be frequently well in excess of this figure – and prefer the stricter figure of 30% recommended in 1983 for the UK population by the National Advisory Committee for Nutrition Education.

Food frequency data show that South Asians (predominantly Punjabi Muslim) in Glasgow eat many high fat foods significantly less often than the general population, though they are as likely to eat butter and more likely to drink full cream milk and (men) eat meat (Williams, Bhopal and Hunt, 1994); their intake of non-diet drinks, confectionary and ice-cream does not differ significantly from that of the general Glasgow population (Bush *et al.*, 1996). The dietary practices and nutritional status of young South Asian adults and the elderly are largely unexplored, though biochemical markers consistent with insulin resistance have been found even in young South Asian females aged 16–45 (Proudler *et al.*, 1996). The omission of the elderly is partly explained by the generally young age profile of British South Asian communities, but as these communities age, the health and nutritional status of their older members will be highlighted. The current review shows the difficulties being experienced by some elderly South Asians.

2. Studies specifically concerned with food choice

Access: economic, material and structural barriers and opportunities

We have described how research relating to the health of South Asians in Britain has focused largely on highly specific sub-groups and conditions. This section shows that evidence for elevated rates of diseases with a potential nutritional basis is frequently interpreted as a consequence of South Asians' linguistic and cultural differences, and seldom in the context of the social disadvantage which derives from generally high unemployment and poor housing (Ahmad, 1989).

This section presents evidence for potential barriers to, and opportunities for, access to food which promotes good nutritional health, taking the data in the sequence of the lifecourse. However, in much of the literature the concern is for access, or the lack of it, to culturally appropriate food rather than to food which is, first and foremost, 'healthy', although these concepts are often felt to overlap. 'Current food policies, where they exist, address the issue of healthy eating generally but not the specific provision of food traditionally eaten by black and ethnic minorities. These foods have a lot to contribute to a healthy diet' (Hill, 1987, p. 33). While this is true, we have tried to draw attention to instances where implications for healthy eating are not necessarily as clear as is assumed.

The greater part of the literature cited is from data-based studies which give varying degrees of detail concerning methodology and sample size. Other sources include the review *Low income, food, nutrition and health: strategies for improvement* (Low Income Project Team, 1996), and reports of meetings of health professionals concerned with dietary prevention of CHD (Falshaw, 1993) and minority ethnic representatives concerned with food provision (Hill, 1987). The latter represents expert opinion without formal data available to refer to.

Barriers and opportunities presented by social class, income or access to food retail outlets

South Asians, particularly Pakistanis and Bangladeshis, tend to have low incomes (see 'Income' in Section 1 above), and the diets of those living on low incomes and in poverty tend to be restricted in variety and nutrients, lowering resistance to a range of diseases found more often in those living in poor economic circumstances (Low Income Project Team, 1996). In addition, some South Asian groups may be doubly disadvantaged, by constraints on access to the particular diet to which they are accustomed as well as by low income.

There is a considerable body of evidence linking dietary fat with CHD (Department of Health, 1994a), and dietary fat consumption has been shown to vary by social class: Bolton Smith and colleagues (1990) report significant differences between non-manual and manual classes for men and women in Scotland. A survey of dietary fat purchasing habits of 'whites, blacks and Asian peoples' in Birmingham (Lip *et al.*, 1995) found a trend to greater amounts of fat in foods bought in social classes IV and V in 'white and Asian' groups (though not significant), but not in the black group, even though blacks were equally likely to be in social class IV–V or unemployed (p. 290). A higher quantity of fat in foods bought per week was found in the Asian population than in the white (NS) and black groups ($p = 0.03$), and butter, egg, milk and ghee consumption and use of frying was greater among Asians. Given the elevated rates of CHD in South Asians in Britain, these findings indicate a serious barrier to nutritional health, but are rendered less useful by a lack of differentiation of South Asian groups, the primary aim being to identify differences between wider ethnic groups (p. 291). Their recommendation that 'the Asian community should be targeted for intense dietary intervention and other preventative measures' (p. 287) must be qualified, given the clear dietary differences between South Asian sub-groups noted in other studies (see below).

Income influences not only the variety and quality of food purchased but also the type and location of food outlet chosen. Moreover, the type of outlet frequently determines the variety and quality of food on sale. Out-of-town superstores, which offer lower prices, greater choice and better quality, are deliberately sited to suit car owners in higher income brackets; those on low incomes and the elderly, who spend more of their income on food, are generally not able to reach them since they usually walk to the shops or take public transport. The burgeoning of superstores in recent years has led to a 35% reduction in food retail outlets in suburban areas, mainly through the loss of specialist shops such as butchers and greengrocers (Low Income Project Team, 1996). It has also contributed in part to the demise of the Asian 'corner shop' (Meikle, 1996), causing economic hardship and potential damage to health through the requirement to work long hours to stay in business. Increasingly, food retail outlets in high streets and low income areas are discount stores or freezer centres which generally stock a limited range and quality, particularly of fresh fruit and vegetables (Meikle, 1996; Henson, 1992), though vegetables are the second largest category of frozen foods in such stores (Low Income Project Team, 1996), and their nutrient quality may be greater than in fresh vegetables which have been picked for some time.

How far South Asians need the Asian corner shop to obtain the full variety of their diet is unclear, as studies of the food purchasing practices of South Asians are few. A small dietary study of Sikh and Muslim women in Glasgow noted that 8 of the 10 subjects used small, local, Asian food stores for 'a sizeable proportion' of their food shopping (Anderson and Lean, 1995, p. 130); 3 of these 8 also used large supermarkets, one used a wholesale outlet and another a department store. Two other women used only large supermarkets except for daily bread and milk which was bought at smaller shops.

Some supermarket chains are now providing free bus services and home deliveries, as well as fresh fruit and vegetables at low prices or in extra value packs (Low Income Project Team, 1996). Such moves may help remove barriers to cheaper foods which some South Asian groups encounter, but in so doing may contribute further to the decline of South Asian food stores. Further, while some supermarkets carry a number of culturally appropriate foods such as pulses, rice and some fruits and vegetables, halal meat and 'traditional' South Asian vegetables are unlikely to be available other than at specialist shops. The Institute of Grocery Distribution carried out three case studies in deprived urban areas; 'in one area with a high proportion of minority ethnic households, access to traditional foods was limited to small local shops' (cited in Low Income Project Team, 1996). South Asian foods have become more available with increased importation, but may be expensive simply because they are imported (Douglas, 1993).

The cost of food may not of course be decisive. In a recent study in Glasgow, migrant South Asian women were more likely than British-born South Asian women, migrant and British-born Italian women, and general population women to say that their food choice would not change given an increase or decrease in income. They also spent a greater proportion of their income on food than did British-born South Asian and general population women, who had similar levels of income (Bush and Williams, 1995). Similarly a survey of South Asians in Central Scotland found that neither availability nor cost was reported as influencing food choice, although these respondents may not be representative (Landman and Wyke, 1995).

Difficulties with providing appropriate quantities and packaging of South Asian foods have been indicated (Hill, 1987). Quantities available in supermarkets may be inappropriate for family catering if, as has been suggested, the custom of bulk buying favoured on the Indian subcontinent is continued in Britain. Conversely, the elderly who do not wish to bulk-buy (Hill, 1987), and have no access to supermarkets, may experience difficulties in obtaining appropriate foodstuffs, which in turn could adversely affect levels of food consumption and ultimately their nutritional status. Bhalla and Blakemore (1981) found 5% of elderly South Asians to be living alone.

Financial necessity leading to a return to work has been offered as a partial explanation for early discontinuation of breast-feeding by 'Asian' (Treuherz, Cullinan and Saunders, 1982) and Pakistani (Griffiths, 1983) women.

Information relating to South Asians of pensionable age is limited, but what data there are indicate that they are likely to be confronted by a number of barriers to nutritional health, including poverty, low use of social services (see next section) and physical incapacity. A literature survey by Mays (1983) led him to suggest that a number of problems with obtaining state pensions will cause elderly South Asians in general to have low personal incomes, and that those who came to Britain as dependents and are thus not eligible for state support will be totally dependent upon their families. In 1979, only 46 per cent of South Asian elderly surveyed in Birmingham were receiving state benefits (Bhalla and Blakemore, 1981). Thus elderly South Asians may be vulnerable to the difficulties which low income presents for food provision and purchase.

An age-related decline in physical capacity may present difficulties in shopping for and preparing food. A survey of primarily Indian-born elderly in the city of Leicester reports that 'over half of the over 75s were not fully independent in basic activities of daily living' (Donaldson, 1986). A sample of North London Gujaratis (mean age 63.9) was found to have significantly lower expiratory flow rates and grip strength than non-South Asians, which could 'lead to premature arrival at age-related thresholds of physical capacity essential for independence in activities of daily living' (Ebrahim *et al.*, 1991).

Barriers and opportunities presented by institutional menus
Information about the food choice of South Asians away from home is particularly limited, and what there is deals chiefly with institutional food. Hill's (1987) report of discussion groups provides some data, notably with regard to the range of circumstances in which South Asians and other minority ethnic groups encounter institutional catering, in schools and hospitals, at luncheon clubs and from Meals-on-Wheels. The latter in particular are greatly underused by South Asians in comparison with the general population (Bhalla and Blakemore, 1981; Ali and Begum, 1991; Atkin and Rollings, 1993; Askham, Henshaw and Tarpey, 1995; Ahmad and Walker, 1997), a cause for concern given the barriers of poverty and physical incapacity confronting some elderly South Asians. Underfunding of the voluntary sector has been said to account for the fact that there is only one luncheon club for Bangladeshis in Tower Hamlets (Ali and Begum, 1991).

Meal provision by social and health authority services for minority ethnic elderly has been reviewed (Askham, Henshaw and Tarpey, 1995). Thirty-eight (62.3%) of 61 social services departments (SSDs) and 39 (66.1%) of 59 district health authorities (DHAs) responded to a postal survey in 1990, with a lower than average response in Greater London. A quarter of SSDs and one in eight DHAs made no specific or separate provision for ethnic minorities in Meals-on-Wheels and hospital catering. Authorities preferred the type of provision in which specific attention is made to ethnic minorities' needs within a general service, rather than a service which is separate from that of the majority, except for day care. Some authorities said they lacked knowledge of South Asian and other ethnic minorities' needs.

Provision by DHAs focused on providing facilities for patients' relatives to cater for them. Although this is undesirable in the long term, not least because it incurs costs for relatives of minority patients which those in the majority do not have to meet, it may be an opportunity for healthy eating on behalf of the patient who might otherwise be inadequately fed while in hospital. In an additional qualitative study appended to the postal survey, eighty-three per cent of 89 South Asians aged 50–75 said special diet would be important to them as patients, one women illustrating the potentially serious consequences of inappropriate food provision: 'I would rather not eat than be forced to eat something I do not like' (Askham, Henshaw and Tarpey, p. 86).

Schools may be seen as detrimental to 'traditional' food practices, because of the prominence of ethnic majority convenience foods, particularly chips which children are said to eat rather than a packed lunch, the ownership of which results in 'harassment and racist comments' (Shukla, in Hill, 1987, p. 4). If these claims could be substantiated, they could indicate a barrier to nutritional health, assuming that the packed lunch is more nutritionally sound than the alternative.

Hill's report also considers catering in the workplace and in hospital. Common to both is the difficulty that, although intended as 'traditional', food may not resemble that which is eaten at home and be rejected; the setting up of 'recipe banks' is proposed to circumvent this. Moreover, since hospital diet is based upon Western nutritional concepts, pre- and post-natal women may be challenged if they follow the Ayurvedic or Unani systems which view pregnancy as a 'hot' condition to be balanced by the consumption of cooling foods (Dobson, 1988); we discuss these beliefs in more detail in the following section. The provision of culturally appropriate food may require considerable negotiation; in Dewsbury it involved consultation with management about catering budgets, in-service training of catering staff, and issues of policy regarding food provided by relatives (Rocheron and Dickinson, 1990). Such complexity could discourage persistence by authorities to introduce appropriate food, and thus could be a barrier to short-term nutritional health.

Culturally appropriate food could be introduced in the workplace, in hospitals and in services used by the elderly through employing members of ethnic minorities, either in paid or voluntary capacities (Hill, 1987), or by contracting out to them (Blakemore and Boneham 1994, p. 134). This could present a valuable opportunity for healthy eating, particularly as it would offer an alternative to the type of foods described by Smith and colleagues (1993) in two factories in Bradford. Although the food choice of South Asian men in the study was less influenced by catering facilities and shift patterns than that of 'Caucasian' men, with home-prepared curry being eaten two or three times a day, some South Asian men reported eating fried egg sandwiches at breaktimes, and foods such as fish and chips, pies and pasties, but whether this was because of a lack of South Asian foods is not reported. Fried foods were consumed with a similar frequency by South Asian and other men, although the former primarily ate samosas and other fried Asian foods, presumably not provided by the canteen. Consumption of culturally appropriate food in this instance does not equate with good nutritional health. Changes in catering at one factory were made as a consequence of involvement in the study although these are not described.

Apart from institutional menus, food other than home-prepared may be consumed in cafés, restaurants and 'fast-food' outlets. Again, little information is available which describes South Asian use of such facilities. A study of food choice in migrant and British-born South Asian women aged 20–40 in Glasgow found that 65% of the former and 34% of the latter never eat in a restaurant.* Sheikh and Thomas (1994b) surveyed South Asian (mainly Gujarati Hindu) and 'Caucasian' teenagers (12–16 years) in a Harrow comprehensive school, and their results indicated the popularity of fast foods with this age group. South Asians, particularly girls, were significantly more likely than others to eat pizza, and this was eaten with families at home and in pizza restaurants, apparently because of the availability of a vegetarian option. More South Asian girls than boys tended to frequent hamburger outlets, but those who did not eat meat opted for chips or a vegetarian burger; however, the outlets, rather than the food on offer, appear to be the focus of interest since they act as a 'meeting-point as part of their social routine' (p. 32). Use of fast-food outlets by young people has been seen as a cause for concern, because of the selection of foods low in nutrients (Department of Health survey, 1989, cited in Sheikh and Thomas), but although Sheikh and Thomas's reporting does not permit assessment of the nutritional impact of fast-food consumption, it does illustrate a considerable appeal of such food for South Asian teenagers and, apparently, their family members.

Barriers and opportunities in access to food information
Frequent reference is made in the literature to issues of information. Lack of appropriate knowledge on the part of health professionals and South Asians, differences in 'traditional' and biomedical opinion, and problems with communicating information, particularly because of language difficulties, are described. Linguistic ability is a recurring theme in reports and descriptions of infant feeding practices particularly, although these tend to involve small numbers of subjects. Because language problems present striking practical difficulties to health professionals they may be assumed rather than demonstrated to be the cause of nutritional problems.

A study of 26 Bangladeshi women in Newcastle identified 'serious language problems in communicating with health professionals' (Shahjahan, 1991, p. 19), with 69% of mothers requiring an interpreter.

*Unpublished data from Dietary Change in South Asian and Italian Women in the West of Scotland, a research project funded by the ESRC as part of 'The Nation's Diet' Research Programme and carried out at the MRC Medical Sociology Unit, Glasgow.

Considerable misunderstanding of information regarding the duration of breast-feeding and type of weaning food was evident, which has been noted elsewhere in this group of women (Wallace, Ahmed and Iqbal, 1992), perhaps because of the number of meetings with health professionals made without interpreters or with the help of family members, sometimes older children (p. 21). Thirty-five per cent of 43 South Asian women (mainly Pakistani) taking part in one study were illiterate (Sahota, 1991), and although their fluency in English is not reported, the finding highlights the importance of oral dissemination of information for such women. In an article on Asian health care, a health visitor hypothesised that language problems may prevent imparting essential information about bottle-feeding to mothers who use this method (Mayor, 1984). She also suggests that health professionals may be unable to give support for breast-feeding mothers which absent family members might otherwise have provided. Burton-Jeangros (1995) sees a similar lack of support from professionals (13 of the 18 women in her survey had not spoken to, or did not remember speaking to, a health professional about feeding practices) but notes this was not peculiar to women without spoken English. Seventy-two per cent of 'Asian' women studied in East London had received information about breast-feeding postnatally, compared to 62 per cent of other women, but only 59 per cent of Asian women reported having 'considerable education on postnatal wards' in contrast to 83 per cent of other women (Woollett et al., 1995, p. 78). Some midwives feel 'uncomfortable' giving dietary advice to women from ethnic minorities and to vegetarians (Mulliner, Spiby and Fraser, 1995, p. 39), but midwives' nutritional knowledge has been reported to be inadequate more generally (Mulliner, Spiby and Fraser, 1995; Wright, 1995).

Information may, of course, come from non-professional sources, and Griffiths (1983, p. 396) suggested that the very low rates of breast-feeding she reports in her study in Birmingham might be due in part to the fact that 'for the Indian and Pakistani mothers the advertisements displaying bonny babies are an additional incentive to bottle-feed'. The number of women who expressed such a view is not documented. Women in Cardiff 'were not very aware of a pressure from the formula milk industry' (Burton-Jeangros, 1995, p. 68).

At the other extreme of the lifecourse, communication difficulties have been proposed as barriers to the use of social services by the elderly. For example, more than half of the 726 South Asians aged 65 and over surveyed in Leicester had not heard of Meals-on-Wheels; less than three per cent were using this service but seven per cent expressed a need for it (Donaldson, 1986). Of South Asians aged 65 and over surveyed in Birmingham only 13 per cent knew of Meals-on-Wheels and only 5 per cent of lunch clubs (Bhalla and Blakemore, 1981). Mays (1983) notes concerns about language difficulties among people not attending day centres, and Bhalla and Blakemore (1981) found 88 per cent of their respondents were unable to speak English.

It may be the content of information, rather than its communication, which constructs barriers. Overcoming language barriers is insufficient, and health professionals should have specific knowledge of food and its social and cultural implications (Samanta et al., 1986). Dietary advice offered in pregnancy may conflict with food practices derived from South Asian systems of medicine. In a small qualitative study of mainly Punjabi women, Homans (1983) reports that some foods prohibited as hot were recommended by allopathic doctors and that vegetarian women were not given appropriate advice. Bhopal (1986a, p. 319) notes that South Asians are poorly informed with regard to health issues, although comparison with the 'indigenous population' in this respect is complicated by the methodological incompatibility of recent studies.

We have described the high prevalence of diabetes in South Asians in Britain, and it has been suggested, unfortunately without substantiation, that a lack of dietary advice hinders good diabetic control (Hawthorne, Mello and Tomlinson, 1993), as does a lack of specificity, possibly stemming from the dietitians' unfamiliarity with South Asian foods (Khajuria and Thomas, 1992). A national questionnaire survey of diabetic clinics with more than 50 South Asians registered found that 40 per cent had no adapted diet sheets (Goodwin, Keen and Mather, 1987). A study of South Asians in Brent (unreferenced in Hill, 1987, p. 36) apparently indicated that the publications of the British Diabetic Association and the Health Education Council do not take account of South Asian diet.

Representatives of ethnic minorities are reported to be critical of nutrition education for children and adults in their ethnic group. It is claimed that information distributed by health authorities is 'often patronising and inappropriately produced' (Hill, 1987, p. 17) because the minorities at whom it is directed are not consulted, and that it portrays minority food as 'tasty' or 'exotic' but fails to emphasise its nutritional value. Some of Landman and Wyke's respondents reported 'ethnocentric' nutrition messages from various sources (1995, p. 61). Further, the emphasis in nutrition education has focused on changing bad habits, rather than acknowledging good ones. While noting again that the strength of this report is undermined by its lack of supporting evidence, its positive attitude to the nutritional value of 'traditional' food suggests a potential receptiveness for more sensitively constructed messages. The belief that South Asian diets are healthy was expressed by 'many adults' in Landman and Wyke's study (1995, p. 46).

We end this section where we began, with poverty, for it may be the low income of some South Asians, rather than a lack of knowledge, which forms a barrier to sound nutritional health: 'coping within a limited food budget is often at the expense of foods known by householders to be "healthier"' (Low Income Project Team, 1996, p. 4). South Asian women (mainly Punjabi and of Punjabi descent) in Glasgow were significantly more likely than general population women to consider low fat foods and high fibre foods as very important (Bush *et al.*, 1995), while 'some women and young people' interviewed in Central Scotland tried to eat salads and to avoid fatty foods (Landman and Wyke, 1995, p. 45), and were keen to eat healthy foods in a South Asian 'style' (p. 66). This suggests the absorption of health education messages.

Culture and food choice

This section discusses barriers and opportunities arising from differences in food choice between groups of South Asians, and between them and the ethnic majority, many of which are associated with the fairly crude forms of ethnic classification which are available, but nothing more, and so represent questions needing explanation. As we have already noted, evidence for elevated rates of diseases with a potential nutritional basis is often viewed as a consequence of South Asians cultural and linguistic differences, and these may be interpreted as deficiencies so that the culture is held to blame. However, there are usually a number of other possibilities as well, and in any case culture is not a stereotyped or rigid phenomenon, so it is important to consider the extent to which evidence of causal pathways is provided.

The majority of the literature focuses on a specific disease or evidence for potential nutritional difficulties, such as rickets, coronary heart disease, diabetes or low birthweight and looks for evidence in the South Asian diet to account for these conditions. There are very few studies of food choice as a whole as an aspect of South Asian culture, including common aspects of health in which it is beneficial.

Barriers and opportunities presented by dietary variation according to religion and migrants' region of origin

We begin with an overview of the principal theoretical dietary differences between South Asian sub-groups before looking at the limited evidence of reported dietary differences. The differential food practices of South Asians stem from their area of origin which determines the staple food and reflects the religious group to which they belong (Sheikh and Thomas, 1994a). The Bangladeshi staple food is rice, and that of Punjabis and Mirpuris from north-west India and Pakistan is wheat, generally taken in the form of chapattis. The staples of Gujaratis in Britain are wheat (Sheikh and Thomas, 1994a) and rice (Shukla, 1991).

South Asians in Britain are primarily followers of the Islamic, Hindu and Sikh faiths, each of which has specific dietary codes which we describe briefly here. South Asian Muslims, followers of the Islamic faith, are primarily from Bangladesh and Pakistan. They follow the dietary rules of the Koran which prohibits pork or pork products and stipulates the consumption of ritually-slaughtered meat which renders it halal. In addition the fast of Ramadan is observed yearly, when for a month no food or drink is taken between dawn and sunset.

Orthodox Hindus are strict vegetarians, rejecting meat, fish, eggs, cheese made with animal rennet, and animal gelatine. The less strict will eat meat, but beef and its products are not eaten since Hindus esteem the cow as sacred; dairy products are permitted, however, because they do not involve the taking of life, and ghee (clarified butter) is believed to sanctify food prepared with it. Milk and yoghurt are also valued (Ganatra, 1989). Pork is thought unclean and generally not eaten (Shukla, 1991). If fish is taken it is usually white (Anon., 1976). Hindus also fast, often to mark religious days; their fasting ranges from total abstention to restriction of quantity and type of food (to those which are considered pure such as milk, fruit, yoghurt, nuts and potatoes).

Lastly, the Sikh religion originates in a reform which sought to combine Muslim and Hindu beliefs in a fresh synthesis. Sikhs have few dietary taboos, but some Sikhs are vegetarian, and beef and pork may also be avoided. Meat, fish and eggs are never served at the regular communal meals in Sikh temples to avoid giving offence to vegetarian Sikhs. Butter and ghee are the most commonly used fats in Sikh cooking, with occasional use of oil (Ganatra, 1989). As this section progresses we will see how some of these dietary practices may present opportunities for, and barriers to, good nutritional health, and how some have been implicated in specific diseases held to be particularly prevalent in South Asians in Britain.

Vegetarianism
This primarily Hindu dietary practice (but one also common to varying degrees among women in all these faiths) has been highlighted in a number of studies. For example, a review of the medical records of South Asian migrants in South London found a higher incidence of tuberculosis among Hindus than among Muslims, and concluded that this might be a consequence of vegetarianism, although no dietary information was available (Finch, Millard and Maxwell, 1991). To obtain such data, a case-control study of TB in immigrant South Asians was carried out (Strachan et al., 1995). This confirmed an increased risk for Hindus, but religion had no independent influence after adjustment for vegetarianism. Vegetarian diet 'appeared to be the main explanation for the Hindu excess' (p. 178). Adjustment for socioeconomic and other variables had little effect on relative risk.

Vegetarian diet was 'the major determinant' of the varying degrees of severity of osteomalacia noted in South Asians in South London, the severity of the disease being associated with increasingly strict dietary practice (Finch *et al.*, 1992). Multivariate analysis showed that being Hindu was a major determinant of vegetarianism. Adherence to a vegetarian diet became less rigid with increasing length of residence in Britain, and it was concluded that while health education 'should perhaps concentrate on those at greatest risk' that is, vegetarians, notably female, changes in the diet over time indicate 'that the problem may eventually disappear'. Vegetarianism was found to be 'strongly related' to osteomalacia in South Asian women in Glasgow (Henderson *et al.*, 1990, p. 923). Those eschewing meat, fish and eggs (Sikh and Hindu in this study) had significantly greater risk than those who simply ate no meat or fish. Of the 13 most severely affected 12 were Sikh or Hindu; the only Muslim in this group had been a strict lactovegetarian from childhood. This tends to support Strachan's finding that it is vegetarianism, rather than religion, which could be identified as a barrier in these studies. No reference is made to rates of osteomalacia in vegetarians in the British ethnic majority which would help to put the South Asian picture into context.

The impact of vegetarian practices on growth of South Asian children in Britain has been explored (Rona *et al.*, 1987). No differences in weight-for-height and triceps skinfolds were found between vegetarians and non-vegetarians; vegetarian girls tended to be shorter than non-vegetarian, but this only approached significance in one group. Unfortunately, this group is classified as 'Urdu'; this is a language rather than a sub-national group, but Urdu-speakers are predominantly from Pakistan.

Others have noted positive aspects of vegetarian diet. For example, using data derived from three separate studies of Punjabi Sikh men and Gujarati Hindu women and men in London, Kassam-Khamis and colleagues (1995) identified a wider range of dishes commonly eaten by the mainly vegetarian Gujaratis in comparison to Sikhs, who ate meat. Smith and colleagues (1993) reported that the Asian men in their study ate a much more varied range of vegetables, including pulses, than did 'Caucasians'; this was particularly true for Hindus because fewer ate meat. Since vegetable consumption tends to be associated with higher intakes of fibre, vitamins and minerals, and dietary variety too is important to achieve an appropriate nutrient intake (Low Income Project Team, 1996), vegetarianism may be an opportunity for good nutritional health in this respect.

As one of a series of studies of 813 pregnant South Asian women in Harrow, Abraham and colleagues (1987) reviewed the diets of 138 Muslims, who ate meat, and 675 Hindus, 450 of whom were vegetarians of varying degrees of strictness. Diets were compared to 54 'European controls'. The women were 'relatively affluent' (Campbell-Brown *et al.*, 1985) and had retained their pre-migration food culture to a large extent (Abraham *et al.*, 1985). South Asians as a whole were found to have lower levels of vitamin D and B12, particularly in the vegetarian groups, but the study concluded that it was 'neither desirable nor necessary to recommend alterations to the Gujarati diet in a community such as this', except for vitamin D supplementation. The authors indicate that their findings are applicable to non-pregnant South Asian women in Harrow since evidence from other studies suggests diets in pregnancy do not change greatly. An earlier study in this series (Abraham *et al.*, 1985) found protein and zinc intakes of South Asians, particularly vegetarians, to be lower than those of controls, but no consequent adverse maternal or foetal consequences were apparent.

The range of potential causes of vitamin D deficiency has given rise to an extensive, and sometimes contradictory, literature concerning rickets and osteomalacia in South Asians in Britain, with religious and cultural practices being implicated. Diet is particularly singled out for blame because of, for example, the absence of vitamin D-rich oily fish in vegetarian diets (Robertson *et al.*, 1982) and the high phytate content of chapatti flour which may indirectly impair vitamin D absorption (Clements, 1989). Dietary modifications have been proposed, such as the total exclusion of chapattis (Ford *et al.*, 1972). More extreme is the belief that the Western diet, high in meat, fish and dairy foods, protects against the deficiency, leading to the conclusion 'that the prevalence of rickets and osteomalacia would be greatly reduced if the Asian population of Great Britain were to adopt such a diet' (Robertson *et al.*, 1982, p. 246). Attempts to persuade South Asians to abandon their traditional diet are undesirable, not simply because of the 'cultural élitism' they imply, which Robertson and her colleagues themselves recognised (1982, p. 147), but also because in important respects the various diets of South Asians are 'generally healthier than that of the native British population' (McKeigue and Chaturvedi, 1996, p. 58). It is, therefore, a matter of concern on both these counts that the notion of dietary adaptation continues to be promulgated (for example Finch *et al.*, 1992; Iqbal *et al.*, 1994).

Inter-group variation

Kassam-Khamis and colleagues (1995) found considerable variation in the fat and energy contents of recipes for comparable dishes. Although intra-group variation was also marked, the mean fat values for Gujarati recipes were often higher than comparable Punjabi recipes, which, according to the authors, might reflect the greater affluence of Gujaratis in Brent and Wembley. The higher fat values are of concern, but the variation is particularly encouraging, for the dishes cooked with less fat must be palatable to those consuming them, so there is potential for the production of lower fat versions of 'traditional' dishes (Kassam-Khamis *et al.*, 1995), assisting individuals to reduce their intake of dietary fat while maintaining a diet they find acceptable.

Variation in nutrient intake and dietary patterns between groups has been observed in studies concerned with South Asian diet in pregnancy (Wharton, Eaton and Wharton, 1984) and as a risk marker for coronary heart disease (Smith *et al.*, 1993). Wharton surveyed Pakistani, Sikh, Hindu and Bangladeshi women in Birmingham. Sikhs were reported to eat the greatest variety of foods, with few eating meat; the Hindu diet was very similar to the Sikh but contained more meat, chicken and rice. This surprising finding may indicate a post-migratory modification of the diet. Bangladeshi women ate a less varied diet, with considerably less fruit being consumed than in the other groups, which the authors suggest could explain their lower levels of vitamin C. Vegetables were also consumed less frequently but, unlike the other groups, Bangladeshis ate fish regularly. They also had lower intakes of fat, possibly because they did not eat paratha or chapatti which are reported as being popular with the other three groups. Pakistani women had vitamin intakes generally greater than Bangladeshis but less than Sikhs and Hindus; vitamin C intakes were good, possibly because of the popularity of fruit in the Pakistani diet. The consequences for health of these differences are not clear (p. 475).

Smith and colleagues' (1993) comparison of South Asian and 'Caucasian' men in Bradford revealed the generally positive effect of their overall adherence to a traditional pattern of food choice, in that the South Asian men ate fresh fruit, salad, lamb, poultry and yoghurt more often, and white fish, processed meat products, chips, potatoes and sweet baked products less often than did Caucasian men. In Glasgow, South Asians ate meat and fruit, salad and raw vegetables more often than the general population, but there were considerable variations by religion (Williams, Bhopal and Hunt, 1994). When the diets of Hindu and Muslim men in Bradford were compared, a number of differences in food patterns were noted, in particular that fats high in saturated fatty acids were used less by Hindus than Muslims, a finding assigned to the former's lower meat intake, greater consumption of vegetables and variations in the uses of fats. Knight *et al.* (1992) also found more meat and fewer vegetables in the diets of Muslims in comparison with Hindus. Not only do these differences have potential health implications, but their recognition is essential if health messages are to be appropriate.

Adherence to these traditional foods is affected by exposure to the ethnic majority culture and by decline in religious observance. Kassam-Khamis, Thomas and Judd (1996) found that having white friends, eating in non-Asian homes, and being born in Britain was associated with reduced consumption of traditional foods and increased consumption of Western foods. The second generation were also less observant of halal prohibitions and of food prescribed for religious festivals. The implications of this obviously vary according to the healthiness of the traditional diet.

Finally in this section we note the varying degrees of adherence to religiously-prescribed food practices by school pupils in Harrow, and also that 30 per cent of boys and 26 per cent of girls did not adhere to any such practices. The primary reason reported was a difference of opinion from that of parents regarding the desirability of religious influence upon daily life, while in other cases respondents followed one or both parents' example of not following the dietary restrictions of their religion, or else they received no opposition to their rejection of them (Sheik and Thomas, 1994b). The rejection of such dietary restrictions and adoption of a more Western diet could have serious health consequences, depending on their degree and extent.

Barriers and opportunities presented by patterns of eating according to gender, age and family processes (including child-rearing practices)

The emphasis on studies of infant feeding practices in this section confirms the bias in research interest and health initiatives directed at South Asians in Britain: ' . . . they are all concerned with child or maternal health and Asian people outside these groups are excluded' (Ahmad, 1989, p. 149). Gender comparisons are limited, and no comparisons of food choice by age-group were identified.

Gender comparisons

Differences in the diets of South Asian men and women (primarily Punjabi Muslims, Sikhs and Hindus) in Glasgow have been noted (Williams, Bhopal and Hunt, 1994, p. 31). Although significances for ethnic rather than gender differences were presented, the data indicate that more women than men eat salads/raw vegetables in summer on a daily basis, eat biscuits three or more times a week, and never eat red meat and eggs. Also in Glasgow, Robertson and colleagues (1982) found South Asian boys to have higher intakes of meat than girls, while Kalka (1988) reported that Gujarati women in Harrow are more likely to avoid meat than are men.

Family patterns

Numerous studies describe the infant feeding practices of South Asians in Britain (Burton-Jeangros, 1995; Griffiths, 1983; Harris *et al.*, 1983; Jones, 1987; McNeil, 1985; Sahota, 1991; Shahjahan, 1991; Treuherz, Cullinan and Saunders, 1982; Warrington and Storey, 1988; Williams, Sahota and Fairpo, 1989). In addition, descriptions and reviews have been published, some of which are unreferenced, forming a more impressionistic level of information (for example Mayor, 1984; McGinn, 1989). Attention has focused on the incidence and prevalence of breast-feeding, on the age at which infants are weaned and the nature of the weaning food. In general, the issues concern changes in Britain from the cultural patterns of prolonged breast-feeding and (it appears) late introduction of solid foods in the Indian sub-continent. Curtailment of breast-feeding is likely to be disadvantageous, but earlier weaning beneficial, though it also introduces problems with weaning foods.

Breast-feeding

Comparison of breast-feeding studies is problematic since many describing incidence and prevalence do not state whether breast-feeding is exclusive or whether other fluids are given. These difficulties are not peculiar to studies of South Asian women. Patterns of breast-feeding by South Asian mothers do not appear to be consistent: for example, in Leeds, Williams, Sahota and Fairpo (1989) found significantly smaller percentages of South Asian (Bangladeshi, Pakistani, Punjabi Sikh and Gujarati) than 'white' women breast-feeding at birth (48% v. 61%, $p = 0.05$) and at 6 months (11% v. 22%, $p = 0.05$); in Bradford percentages of Asian (93% Pakistani and Bangladeshi Muslims) and 'European' mothers who breast-fed initially were virtually the same (44% v. 45%), although an additional 14% of Asian mothers used a mix of breast- and bottle-feeding initially (Sahota, 1991). In a survey of 18 Pakistani women (one of whom was British-born) in Cardiff, all but one (who was taking medication) initiated breast-feeding, but only seven babies were exclusively breast-fed at 4 weeks (Burton-Jeangros, 1995). McNeil (1985) found only 8% of 80 Punjabi women in the UK exclusively breast-feeding at 6 weeks, considerably fewer than in findings by Harris and colleagues (1983) showing approximately 50% of Bangladeshi women in Tower Hamlets exclusively breast-feeding at 4 weeks, and a little over 40% at eight weeks. McNeil (1985) reports that the 80 babies studied in the Punjab received breast milk exclusively from birth until an average age of 5 months. To set these findings in context, in 1980, 41% of babies in Britain were receiving some breast milk at 6 weeks (Passmore and Eastwood, 1986, p. 579), but this fell to 38% by 1985 (White et al., 1992); figures for exclusive breast-feeding are not available.

The balance of this evidence is for a turning-away from the breast-feeding practices of the Indian sub-continent, and this is confirmed by the most recent and comprehensive study, for a sample from areas covering 95% of the South Asian population living in England, which shows that higher proportions of mothers in South Asian groups than white mothers from the same areas had breast-fed during the first week, but higher proportions also gave up at ages up to 8 weeks, gradually extinguishing the differences and, in the case of Pakistani babies, resulting in lower proportions than white babies being breast-fed between 5 weeks and 9 months (Thomas and Avery, 1997). Evidence from mothers born outside the UK indicated that 30–40% who had never breast-fed or had stopped by the first interview would have breast-fed longer or breast-fed entirely if the baby had been born in the mother's native country. Fewer South Asian mothers breast-fed immediately, and mothers who breast-fed immediately were less likely to stop than those who waited more than 24 hours. Sahota (1991, p. 10) cites earlier DHSS data which indicate delays in initiating breast-feeding are associated with its early cessation. She found 24% of South Asian women delayed for between two to five days, and suggests that this reflects the 'traditional' practice of withholding colostrum (a fluid, rich in protein, fat and antibodies, which is expressed in the days after birth before milk itself is produced) since it is held to be unclean. Without help from the mother-in-law or other supportive women the mother may have difficulty establishing feeding after a delay (Sahota, 1991).

Other factors governing the variable degree of change are unclear. One suggestion was that local economic difficulties forced women to work soon after giving birth, so that baby-care was shared with their families, presumably making breast-feeding impracticable (Treuherz, Cullinan and Saunders, 1982). This issue was apparently not raised with mothers, but economic reasons for discontinuing breast-feeding have been reported in Pakistani women in Birmingham (Griffiths, 1983). However, few studies give subjects' employment details, and in those that do working women are in the minority. Early discontinuation of breast-feeding or initial failure to breast-feed may stem from a misunderstanding of advice (Shahjahan, 1991) or lack of support from health professionals or from the absence of experienced family members. In an informal description of a study examining child-rearing practices of South Asians in 1950s Pakistan and 1980s Britain, McGinn (1989) argues that valuable information and support about breast-feeding, which at one time would have been passed down the generations, is being lost. McGinn makes a strong plea for health professionals and the Asian community to recognise 'that it is possible to adapt old ways to new situations, and not discard everything that was of value' (p. 125).

Weaning

Most authors interpret this as the introduction of solid foods. The current recommendation is that 'the majority of infants should not be given solid foods before the age of four months' (Department of Health, 1994b), replacing a recommendation for their gradual introduction, preferably not before 3 months and not later than 6 (Nutrition Standing Committee of British Paediatric Association, 1988). In Leeds Pakistani, Punjabi Sikh and Gujarati women introduced solids at an average age of 4–5 months in all groups, while Bangladeshi women did so at an average age of 6–7 months, and with the greatest age range, between 1 month to more than a year (Williams, Sahota and Fairpo, 1989). Eighty-seven per cent of Bangladeshi babies surveyed in Tower Hamlets received some solids by 6 months, but there was an even greater range for their introduction of 2 months to 2 years, and a tendency for later weaning in mothers who had lived in Britain for less than three years (Harris *et al.*, 1983). In a much smaller study of Bangladeshi women in Tower Hamlets, Jones (1987) found the introduction of solids at 6 months or older by 48% of women, though no 'Caucasian' women did so after 6 months. Eighty-one per cent of 26 Bangladeshi woman surveyed in Newcastle started solids between 3 and 5 months, and the remaining 19% between 6 and 8 months (Shahjahan, 1991). In Bradford South Asian and other women generally introduced solids between 2 and 6 months, but 17% of non-South Asians did so at 1 to 2 months, considerably in advance of the recommended age, whereas only 5% of South Asians did so; 3% of South Asians waited until 6 to 9 months (Sahota, 1991). In Birmingham, solid food was given to Indian babies at $7\frac{1}{2}$ months on average, and to Pakistani babies at $9\frac{1}{2}$ months (Griffiths, 1983). Warrington and Storey (1988b) report 14% of South Asian women introducing solid food at 3 months (compared to 46% of 'Caucasians'), with an average time of 14 weeks, which they indicate is earlier than would have occurred on the Indian sub-continent, citing comparable findings of Aykroyd and Hossain (1967) and Goel (1979). McNeill (1985) reports Punjabi infants in Britain being introduced to solids at an average age of 4 months, compared to $7\frac{1}{2}$ months in the Punjab. On balance, South Asian women in these studies introduced solid foods later than recommended, and their delay may reflect established South Asian practices which do not include a gradual weaning with cereal and then more varied solids (Sahota, 1991), although use of baby cereal was noted by South Asians other than Bangladeshis in Leeds (Williams, Sahota and Fairpo, 1989). The more recent studies of Williams and of Shahjahan indicate solid foods are given at a time more comparable to the recommendation, suggesting a positive change in this aspect of infant feeding practice. This is borne out by the most recent figures on weaning, which show that by 4 months over 90% of all South Asian groups had introduced solid food (Thomas and Avery, 1997).

Weaning foods

The use of commercial weaning foods by South Asian mothers (Harris *et al.*, 1983; Jones, 1987; Sahota, 1991; Shahjahan, 1991; Warrington and Storey, 1988b) is a cause for concern because of their low protein and iron content (Harris *et al.*, 1983). Commercial foods may also be less energy-dense than home-prepared, energy being the main requirement at weaning (Nutrition Standing Committee of British Paediatric Association, 1988). Mothers may not feed 'traditional' foods to infants because they are unsure how to modify them (Mayor, 1984), but solids given to babies in the Punjab are primarily selected from the usual family diet, with potato, chappati, dhal and yoghurt, for example, being given in small amounts (McNeill, 1985). If uncertainty lies behind the absence of 'traditional' foods for weaning, it may be further indication of a lack of influence of the older generation and absence of information concerning established practices.

Use of sweet commercial weaning foods seems particularly prevalent among Bangladeshis, and some reports suggest it may be because savoury baby foods are not halal and are therefore unacceptable to Muslim women. Some mothers are suspicious of vegetarian meals because meat or meat extracts may been used in the manufacturing process (Sahota, 1991).

We note the paucity of studies concerning the infant feeding practices of Hindu women. The focus on Bangladeshis in particular is likely to stem from their perceived vulnerability in terms of health status, physical environment and socioeconomic circumstances. The most recent figures continue to suggest a narrower range of solid food is given to Bangladeshi babies (Thomas and Avery, 1997). In the last decade or so the overall rate of breast-feeding in Britain has increased but babies in low income households are less likely to be breast-fed (Low Income Project Team, 1996); thus the low frequency of breast-feeding in South Asian groups may simply reflect their more constrained socioeconomic position (Aukett and Wharton, 1989). Studies of Hindu women, who are generally in considerably more favourable circumstances, could differentiate between socioeconomic position and culture as influences on infant feeding practices.

Family eating patterns

Aside from infant feeding practices, there are some limited data on family eating patterns. A small study of Sikh and Muslim migrant women in Glasgow indicated the importance of the main evening meal, both in nutritional and social terms, since it constitutes the greater part of daily food intake and is particularly likely to consist of home-made dishes of the South Asian cuisine (Anderson and Lean, 1995). This presents an opportunity for good nutritional health for, although convenience foods of the majority culture are consumed, particularly at lunch-time, many important features of the South Asian diet are retained while, at the same time, 'healthier' versions of basic foods, such as reduced fat milk, have been adopted.

An impressionistic report of a survey of Gujarati migrants in Harrow also reveals the importance of serving the main meal in the evening, so that all family members can eat together (Kalka, 1988). Since migration this meal has been modified from two courses to one, perhaps because the women have less time for cooking than in Gujarat, although 'some Gujaratis' mentioned the need to control the amount of food consumed; the latter may reflect the influence of Hindu religious beliefs upon dietary practice.

Barriers and opportunities presented by other beliefs, values, knowledge, norms and attitudes

The Ayurvedic and Unani medical systems emphasise the role of food in the causation, prevention and treatment of disease, especially as part of the 'hot/cold' theory of nutrition and disease (Bhopal, 1986b). These systems exist side-by-side with Western medicine in the Indian sub-continent, and are maintained by South Asians in Britain, although to what extent is not certain. From his survey of South Asians in Glasgow, Bhopal (1989a, p. 319) concluded that 'Asians seem to accept Western health concepts without difficulty', and that their health beliefs do not interfere with health promotion.

The pre- and postnatal nutritional recommendations which are part of South Asian health belief systems have been proposed, on slight evidence, to explain poor maternal weight gain and low birthweight. Pregnancy is viewed as a 'hot' state so that 'hot' foods such as meat, fish, eggs, some pulses and numerous other foods are avoided in favour of 'cool' foods, notably dairy products, with the potential for protein deficiency, although Bhopal (1986a) suggests specific South Asian dietary practices cannot be held to account for reported poor maternal diet and adverse birth outcomes. Some of the literature on maternal and infant nutrition and health conveys the view that South Asian health beliefs are inherently erroneous and as such must be eradicated and replaced by Western allopathic beliefs. Woollett and colleagues (1995) report the influence of 'cultural beliefs and practices' (p. 65) on South Asians' ideas about diet in pregnancy, but advocate their consideration rather than outright rejection, recommending the education of antenatal staff to this end.

Woollett (1995) found more South Asian women than others to be restricted in cooking and leaving the home following childbirth; the former tended to attribute this to cultural and religious reasons, while the latter tended to offer lack of time or interest as an explanation for these restrictions.

Fasting is another practice associated with South Asian cultures and religions which is hypothesised in the literature as problematic in the context of pregnancy and diabetes, with little evidential support. Indian women may fast in pregnancy to be blessed with a male child (Raman, 1988) or during the last month to discourage foetal growth in order to have an easier delivery (Way, 1991), but the literature gives no clue as to the prevalence of such behaviours in Britain. Better documented is the question whether the fast of Ramadan has any impact on Muslims' health. Fowler and colleagues (1990) retrospectively analysed antenatal clinic attendance during Ramadan in 1989 and for a similar period outside Ramadan. The period of fasting was not seen to have any effect on clinic attendance. A further 78 women were asked about their observation of the fast during pregnancy; of the 82% who said they would fast 56% would do so during pregnancy. Forty-one women believed their calorie intake would be less than normal at this time. Fowler concludes that pregnant Muslims should be encouraged to use their exemption from fasting in Ramadan because of possible adverse consequences of not doing so for their own health and that of their baby. However, Cross and colleagues (1990) reviewed the birthweights of more than 13 000 Muslim babies born in Birmingham over a twenty-year period concluding that the fast of Ramadan has no effect on full-term babies' birthweight at whatever stage of pregnancy it occurred.

The consequences of the Ramadan fast for people with non-insulin-dependent diabetes has been considered in two small studies of Muslims (Beshyah, Jowett and Burden, 1992; Chandalia and Bhargav, 1987), neither finding contra-indications to fasting at this time. In a short review of the practice Rashad (1992) reached a similar conclusion, but notes the need for greater information generally regarding the clinical impact of fasting because of the many millions who observe Ramadan.

McKeigue and Chaturvedi (1996) suggest this time of fasting could be an opportunity for weight loss, but note that fasting is not a long-term solution. That 43% of migrant South Asian women surveyed in Glasgow associated a BMI greater than 28 with eating healthy food may indicate a barrier to weight loss, but evidence for British-born South Asians suggests such views are less common (Bush et al., 1995).

Dietary control is an important element in the management of non-insulin-dependent diabetes, so it is important for advice about food choice to be incorporated into the patient's lifestyle (Kelleher and Islam, 1994). As with all encounters between lay practice and clinical advice, discrepancies occur. The food choice of the 40 South Asians surveyed in a general practice diabetic clinic in Leicester did not correspond to recommendations for diabetic diets, particularly in terms of sweet foods and fats (Samanta et al., 1986). 'A few' felt that the dietary advice they received was not appropriate to their lifestyle and not relevant to the type of food they ate (p. 283). More than half of the Gujarati Hindu vegetarians in a small study in London felt similarly, but all believed food was very important in diabetic control and most understood their diet sheets although 75% had little or no spoken English. Eighty-nine per cent had reduced their fat intake since diagnosis but primarily in terms of restricting visible fat rather than in limiting cooking fat, and the amount of sweet biscuits and gur (sugar) in pickles, curries and pulses indicates the idea of hidden sugar may be unfamiliar (Khajuria and Thomas, 1992). Ample fat or oil in cooking was regarded as necessary to give food the right flavour and physical overweight was held to be indicative of affluence (Samanta et al., 1986), a view observed in 'developing' societies where food supplies are scarce or erratic (Sobal and Stunkard,

1989) but not the predominant view of migrant Punjabi women in Glasgow, who associated overweight, not with economic success but with good health (Bush *et al.*, 1996).

Food plays an essential role in hospitality, and in maintaining the honour of one's family (Bradby, 1996; Bush *et al.*, 1998), and there may be social pressures to eat foods which are contra-indicated for diabetes (Samanta *et al.*, 1986); some Bangladeshis in Tower Hamlets reported being able to resist, but others could not (Kelleher and Islam, 1994). Food's religious connotations may also make them harder to restrict or renounce, as Kelleher and Islam note for Bangladeshis with regard to rice. Ghee is seen as purificatory by Hindus, and since it is also believed to be cooling, soothing, a source of strength and an aid to nutrient absorption, the Western idea that it may be detrimental to health may be a difficult concept for some South Asians (Khajuria and Thomas, 1992). However, that they do partly restrict its intake indicates that this barrier is not insurmountable.

Some vegetables integral to South Asian cuisine are known to reduce blood sugar levels and so may aid diabetic control. These include kerala (Aslam and Stockley, 1979) and fenugreek (Sharma, cited in Kelleher and Islam, 1994). Sixty-four per cent of Gujarati Hindus with diabetes ate vegetables such as these regularly every week or fortnight (Khajuria and Thomas, 1992), and most of the Bangladeshis surveyed by Kelleher and Islam ate kerala. Thus South Asians with diabetes may have opportunities to assist in the dietary management of their disease in ways which are familiar and acceptable to them.

Korlipara (1995) offers a less positive view of dietary management of diabetes. In an unreferenced, personal assessment he states that it is 'unrealistic for doctors to expect elderly patients, especially Asian where cultural and religious considerations need to be taken into account, significantly to alter their diet. Food likes and dislikes are well-entrenched at this age'. Moreover he believes that older people will feel they should be able to indulge their culinary desires, which will outweigh the perceived benefits of major dietary change. He advocates 'earlier pharmacological intervention' for the elderly, rather than dietary therapy alone.

Interventions with South Asians
Coronary heart disease
A plan for health promotion specifically aimed at reducing coronary heart disease has noted the prominent role of primary care (McKeigue and Sevak, 1994), which might be aided by the high proportion of members of ethnic minorities registered with a GP, even in inner-city areas where registration is less common (McKeigue and Chaturvedi, 1996). In a Leeds general practice, 26 per cent of patients attending a

clinic for screening for CHD risk factors in its first 18 months were South Asians, although they made up only 12 per cent of the target population (South, 1993). The high attendance is attributed to the services of an interpreter who is well-known in the local community. Dietary advice, including preferable type and quantity of fat, was given and an increase in the number of families reducing fat in cooking and changing to vegetable oil was noted. 'Several patients' lost weight and 'a lot' of women wanted to lose weight but had difficulty reconciling this with family eating patterns, although this is also true for the majority culture (p. 10), as were other reasons explaining failure to take up advice, such as 'family commitments, habit, health beliefs, environment' and finances (p. 10).

A more extensive primary care initiative has been set up in Tower Hamlets, East London. The Healthy Eastenders Project (Falshaw, 1993) involves the staff of 17 GP practices working to common protocols with a view to prevention of CHD and specific cancers. They have undertaken training to take diet histories and to give dietary advice appropriate to three groups of minority ethnic patients, including Bangladeshi. Working with local communities they have produced health education material to replace existing inappropriate information which made little reference to CHD. They stress the importance of looking beyond the individual to influences on diet at community level such as food availability, poverty and other barriers which prevent people from eating the healthy diet they desire. This led them to consider possible interventions with manufacturers, wholesalers, retailers and distributors, although these are not described, other than the desirability of setting up food co-operatives which allow reduction in food costs through bulk buying. Specific advice for making necessary adaptations to the essentially healthy Bangladeshi diet is also presented, including reduced-fat cooking methods, oily fish which can be substituted for those unobtainable in Britain, and packed lunches for workers and schoolchildren. No evaluation of this intervention was described.

Two randomised control trials awaiting publication have been carried out on South Asians and Europeans in London to determine the feasibility and impact of weight loss (20% body fat) upon risk factors for CHD and diabetes. The first compared the efficacy of dieting and of exercise in 55 South Asians (90% Punjabi Sikhs) aged 35–54, while the second was a dietary intervention in younger men and women (L. Sevak, personal communication, 1996).

Rickets and osteomalacia
The late 1970s and early 1980s saw a number of interventions and evaluative studies which focused on rickets, but these have been generally small and not randomised controlled trials (Peach, 1984). The DHSS/Save the Children Fund Stop Rickets Campaign was intended to

raise South Asians' knowledge of rickets and osteomalacia and of the role of vitamin D through the medium of Asian organisations and health authorities. It aimed at a non-random sample of South Asians, testing knowledge of rickets in a control group, in a second group immediately after receipt of information, and one year later in a third group. Knowledge was greater in the second group than in the other two, but baseline knowledge of rickets in all three groups was not known (Peach, 1984). The campaign has been criticised by Dunnigan and colleagues (1985) for failing to co-ordinate and implement preventive measures. Ahmad (1989, p. 149) is critical because of the campaign's focus on health education, which he believes strongly 'is essentially about culture and victim blaming without due reference to the social circumstances of the sufferers'. However, the campaign did emphasise the benefits of the South Asian diet, and the imbalance which can result from attempts to adopt Western-style eating patterns.

A health education campaign to improve the vitamin D status of South Asians in Rochdale followed a survey in 1970 which revealed overt rickets and osteomalacia within that population (Stephens, Klimiuk and Warrington, 1981; Stephens et al., 1982). Publicity was engendered by the survey, and through subsequent use of posters and leaflets in South Asian shops and meeting places which explained the value of sunlight and consumption of margarine. Health professionals reinforced these messages as the opportunity arose. In this survey and a follow-up in 1980, the South Asians were recruited by self-referral to specially arranged clinics with the encouragement of their community and religious leaders. In the follow-up, the diets of 150 adults and 103 children, chiefly Muslim, were assessed. Despite an increased use of margarine, there was no significant change in the average daily consumption of vitamin D by adults (estimated from seven-day recall), and the 'statistically significant improvement in children is irrelevant in practical terms' (Stephens et al., 1982, p. 442). Further, no significant difference in plasma vitamin D was found between those who ate chapattis and those who did not, nor between meat eaters and 'abstainers'. The health education campaign was deemed to have failed in adults, and the increase in children was insufficient. Dietary advice in the context of vitamin D deficiency was still seen as important, but it was felt unlikely that advice to eat more vitamin D rich foods would be implemented or reduce the prevalence of deficiency.

In an assessment of the efficacy of dietary advice in Southall, 11 South Asian women were counselled on the need to eat vitamin D-rich foods, and compared to an uncounselled control group of nine (Box, 1983). Three separate interviews were conducted with the study group, at which women were asked to recall advice given at previous interviews, which was then reinforced. Mothers-in-law were encouraged to attend, and clinic receptionists used as interpreters when necessary. Reported dietary vitamin D increased in the counselled group only; plasma vitamin D increased in both groups, but the controls showed a greater increase. Falsification of reported dietary change by the counselled group was excluded. It was concluded that although the women could be persuaded to change their diets, the time and effort required was unrewarded by a concomitant increase in plasma vitamin D. Rather, health education messages should focus on using vitamin supplements and increasing South Asians' exposure to sunlight.

Finally, the Glasgow Asian Rickets Campaign, launched in 1979, aimed to reduce the prevalence of rickets through the distribution of free vitamin D supplements on demand to children up to the age of 18, through schools, health centres and selected schools (Dunnigan et al., 1985). A reduction in prevalence was reported two and three years after the start of the campaign in children taking the equivalent of 100 IU of vitamin D daily. Conversely, a health education campaign in Glasgow (1984–86) which promoted vitamin D supplementation to prevent osteomalacia in South Asian women was not successful (Henderson et al., 1989).

Health education campaigns have had little success in changing dietary practice, and it has been shown elsewhere that knowledge alone does not change behaviour (O'Reilly and Shelley, 1991). Correlation studies suggest that the amount of phytate or chapatti in the diet might be more important aetiologically than sunlight or dietary vitamin D (see earlier sub-section on vegetarianism), and since chapatti are central to the diet this supports supplementation as a more effective measure than health education (Peach, 1984). The fortification of foodstuffs with vitamin D, specifically chapatti flour (Singleton and Tucker, 1978), has been recommended (Dunnigan et al., 1985); this would not necessitate dietary adaptation, but was rejected by the COMA Working Party (1980), because of variation in consumption which might cause ineffective or harmful amounts of vitamin D to be ingested. Currently over twice as many South Asian compared with white mothers give vitamin supplements to their babies (Thomas and Avery, 1997). An effective alternative policy to recommending supplements to prevent vitamin D deficiency in South Asians is still awaited (Iqbal et al., 1994).

Maternal and infant health

The Asian Mother and Baby Campaign was funded by the DHSS and designed in partnership with the Save the Children Fund. It ran from September 1984 until March 1986 in 16 health districts with the overall aim of improving the health and well-being of South Asian women and their babies (Rocheron and Dickinson, 1990). Specific aims included the improvement of communication between mothers and health professionals, familiarisation of South Asian families with available services and ensuring services provided are accessible and acceptable

(Bahl, 1987). The campaign had two main features: a programme of publicity and health promotion, and the employment of South Asian women fluent in English and at least one Asian language as linkworkers 'to overcome cultural and linguistic barriers between health professionals and patients'.

The campaign's impact was assessed quantitatively and qualitatively in Dewsbury, Wandsworth and Brent (Rocheron and Dickinson, 1990) and reported extensively (Rocheron and Dickinson, 1990; Rocheron, Dickinson and Khan, 1988; 1989a; 1989b; 1989c). The political and racial issues it evoked have been discussed (Rocheron, 1988). Here we describe findings which may overcome barriers noted in the sections on 'Access' and 'Culture' above. The publicity campaign had limited success, although the use of local media and activities as opposed to national media was felt to have been appropriate, given the popularity of the former with South Asians surveyed in the assessment. Success might have been greater if it had not been assumed that all South Asians required more or similar information (Rocheron and Dickinson, 1990). The lack of definition of linkworkers has been criticised but patients with access to them appear to have enjoyed greater continuity of care, better communication with health professionals, access to detailed information on a range of topics, emotional support and less stress (Rocheron and Dickinson, 1990). Other benefits of the campaign included health education leaflets about local services in relevant languages and more appropriate hospital food. Training sessions for health staff about service delivery to minority ethnic women were also instigated.

Dietary survey/health education methodologies

An exercise with Bengali women in Tower Hamlets tested the extent to which foods were identifiable in pictures intended for use in health education programmes, and whether 'messages' were carried by pictures (Tauber et al., 1980). Forty-four per cent of the woman in the study could not read. Bananas, milk, grapes, aubergine, boiled eggs (photographs), an apple and banana (line drawing) and a woman breast-feeding were identified correctly by 80 per cent of women, but photographs of cooked mince, curry and rice, and carrots were recognised by less than half. Carrots were identified as radishes by 39 per cent of respondents; carrots are luxury vegetables in Bangladesh and radishes tend to be carrot-shaped. The study concluded that unfamiliar objects without verbal explanations are not likely to be recognised, and that pictures may not convey messages without verbal reinforcement. These findings have implications for dietary surveys since photographs of foods may be used to estimate quantities consumed as a more straightforward alternative to weighing.

3. Looking to the future

Socioeconomic trends in South Asians, and the likely impact upon patterns of food choice

Two areas of socioeconomic trends which are particularly relevant to food choice are household structure and income. The notion of the breakdown of 'traditional' living patterns has been challenged (see sub-section on age and gender structure in Section 1), but there is a small amount of evidence which indicates possible change in the circumstances of elderly South Asians. A small inter-regional study reported 13% of elderly South Asians living alone, an increase on earlier studies (Askham, Henshaw and Tarpey, 1995), and unsupported claims for increasing numbers of Bangladeshi elderly living alone in Tower Hamlets have also been made (Ali and Begum, 1991). Although only 5 per cent of elderly South Asians surveyed in Birmingham lived alone, compared to 38% of 'Europeans', 26% had no family in Britain (Bhalla and Blakemore, 1981, p. 15). Mays (1982, p. 78) points to 'limited evidence of changing attitudes to family patterns', specifically from the Community Relations Commission study of 1976, in which more than half of the children in families surveyed said they hoped to live in nuclear families. While the 1991 Census cannot predict the extent to which British-born ethnic minorities will adopt the household patterns of the majority (Murphy, 1996), an increase in the number of elderly living alone or unsupported would be a cause for concern, given the potential barriers to their nutritional health just described.

The 1988–1990 Labour Force Survey and later LFS Quarterly Bulletins show the continued disadvantage of Pakistanis and Bangladeshis in respect of income and employment status, in comparison to Indian people (Jones, 1993; Church and Summerfield, 1996). Two specific examples indicate the potential for continued disadvantage in these groups. On the basis of his recent studies of Bangladeshis in Tower Hamlets, Eade (1989, p. 305) believes the rapidly-growing third generation faces an uncertain economic future which is attributed to competition for jobs and housing with 'white outsiders'. Brah and Shaw (1992, p. 52) conclude that young Muslim women in Birmingham face an uncertain future because of the fundamental changes in the labour market, with the decline in the semi-skilled and unskilled factory jobs which South Asian women previously held, and an increase in low status part-time jobs and 'homeworking', many of which 'lack full social protection'.

Low income and poverty are known to affect diet, but the relationship between these two variables is complicated somewhat by the suggestion that for some South Asians cost does not determine food choice (Landman and Wyke, 1995). We noted earlier that migrant South Asian women in Glasgow were more likely than other women surveyed to say that their food choice would not change given an increase or decrease in income (Bush and Williams, 1995).

Trends in marketing and retailing and the likely impact upon patterns of food choice

No material on these topics peculiar to ethnic minorities was found. An earlier section of this review described the impact which changes in retailing, particularly the development of the supermarket system and the decline of small specialist shops, could have upon food choice of South Asians.

4. Research and intervention priorities

At the beginning of this review we noted the haphazard nature of research interest in South Asian diet, reflecting questions pursued by particular medical specialties on their own account. It is thus important at this point to reconsider the overall seriousness of the health risks involved in the nutritional issues under discussion.

1. Recommendations for general health are represented in the COMA reports. These cover the whole range of diet-related conditions, but the overall benefit from interventions intended to approximate more closely to these recommendations is hard to assess and needs to be the subject of research. These interventions are considered first, but only because of their general scope.

2. Coronary heart disease as the cause of some hundreds of excess premature deaths in the South Asian community per annum (Balarajan and Bulusu, 1990), is clearly a priority, and relevant interventions come next. The probability that *obesity* is closely related to this problem puts it also high on the list.

3. Conditions possibly related to vegetarianism. Vegetarianism may be related to tuberculosis with double figures of excess premature deaths in the South Asian community per annum, to rickets and osteomalacia, painful and disabling conditions of children with implications for adult disability, and to iron deficiency.

4. Infant health and infant feeding practices. The general health of infants and iron deficiency in particular may be affected by aspects of breast-feeding and weaning, though there do not seem to be serious long-term effects on growth (Warrington and Storey, 1988b; Duggan *et al.*, 1992, p. 199).

Our suggestions under these heads are in three main divisions: 1. those identifying potential interventions, 2. those identifying how better to deliver those interventions, and 3. those identifying research priorities.

Practical suggestions on potential interventions
General health
Low income and retail access
- Food co-operatives may be a means of providing cheaper, local, 'traditional' foodstuffs to the numerous South Asian low income groups, bearing in mind the logistical difficulties enumerated by the Low Income Project Team (1996) and the potential for a detrimental impact on South Asian shops; alternatively measures to encourage self-employment in low income areas should be considered as ways of promoting cheap and appropriate food supply through South Asian shops and reducing unemployment.

Institutional menus
- Programmes to facilitate good nutritional health should be community-wide, reaching home and workplace (Smith *et al.*, 1993) or school.

- The use of recipe banks in hospitals, schools and factories should be piloted to determine their value in providing meals which are culturally and nutritionally acceptable. The potential for centralised computer storage and access should be explored.

- Social service departments and district health authorities which currently make no specific provision for South Asians should be encouraged to do so as a 'matter of urgency' and should recognise the range of dietary requirements (Askham, Henshaw and Tarpey, 1995, p. 109).

Access to food information
- Support greater use of health advocates in liaison with dietitians, or of South Asian dietitians trained in health advocacy, whose role would go beyond interpreting, and explanation of health professionals' views to the patient, to representing the patient's understanding of the situation and requirements to health professionals. Many of the studies cited in this review have been conspicuous for the absence of any data on the patient's rationale for relevant behaviours.

Coronary heart disease and control of obesity
- Encourage a reduction in fat used for cooking, since this is the most feasible way of reducing fat intake in South Asians (McKeigue and Chaturvedi, 1996):

  by reducing fat content of staple dishes

  by encouraging the measurement of cooking oil, rather than free-pouring, to increase awareness of how much is used (Carlson, 1993).

- Build on evidence which shows the adoption of reduced-fat alternatives to butter and full-fat milk.

- Encourage Bangladeshi communities to maintain their high fish consumption, since this seems to protect against CHD (McKeigue and Chaturvedi, 1996).

- Work with the trend towards consumption of 'fast' foods and 'take-aways' by encouraging the production of healthier versions (McKeigue and Chaturvedi, 1996).

Conditions possibly related to vegetarianism

- The balance of benefit in vegetarian diets, especially for heart disease, needs to be recognised and preserved in the design of interventions related to vegetarianism. It needs to be acknowledged that both vegetarian and meat eating diets carry risks of excess and deficiency at the extremes. However, there is scope for further design of specific interventions to increase deficient vitamin D and iron intakes at crucial periods, e.g. in pregnancy and childhood, making use of the cultural recognition of these periods as having special dietary requirements in South Asian health beliefs. There may also be scope, if current speculations about the role of vitamin D in tuberculosis are correct, for special interventions in circumstances of particular susceptibility to the disease.

Infant health and infant feeding practices

- Encourage breast-feeding soon after birth, and the use of colostrum, recognising cultural differences and possible tensions which may be created between women who wish to do so and their relatives who may hold other views.

- Discourage pasteurised whole cows' milk as the main milk until after the first twelve months (Department of Health, 1994b).

- Encourage introduction of solids after 4 months and mixed diet by 6 months (Department of Health, 1994b).

- Discourage sweet commercial foods and promote use of South Asian foods for weaning.

- Investigate the feasibility of commercial halal baby food (Shahjahan, 1991; Sahota, 1991).

- Investigate feasibility of labelling commercial weaning foods as halal or suitable for vegetarians in English and South Asian scripts, together with an appropriate symbol for those unable to read.

Enhancing the design of future dietary intervention strategies
General health
Dietary information and health promotion material should:

● differentiate between South Asian sub-groups because of the differences in dietary patterns

● reinforce the essentially healthy nature of South Asian diets (McKeigue and Chaturvedi, 1996), to encourage the retention of positive 'traditional' dietary practices and to counter negative messages which may have discouraged their use; this is especially important for information directed at children and young people, bearing in mind that the healthy nature of food may not be a priority for them

● be readily available and accessible in terms of appropriate and accurate translation; where possible, provision should be made for the effective oral dissemination of information for those unable to read.

Coronary heart disease and control of obesity
● Target South Asian groups appropriately:

reducing total fat is probably more important than changing the type of fat so programmes aimed at the ethnic majority, which emphasise saturated fat, are not generally applicable to South Asians (McKeigue and Chaturvedi, 1996)

the type of dietary fat used also differs between South Asian sub-groups; Gujarati Hindus, for example, have low saturated fat intake (and low plasma cholesterol levels) compared to Punjabi Muslims, to whom advice to substitute unsaturated for saturated fat is more applicable (McKeigue and Chaturvedi, 1996).

● Target young people as well as adults known to be at high risk, as susceptibility to insulin resistance is common outside those known to medical services, and food habits may later be entrenched.

● Interventions to reduce central fat deposition need to include arrangements for monitoring long-term maintenance of the regime, in order to find ways of avoiding harmful swings in fat deposition. They also need to build in use of health advocacy along the lines indicated above under 'Practical suggestions on potential interventions', so as to adapt regimes to individual and family circumstances.

● Interventions should recognise that health is not always the first priority in food choice, and that hospitality, reputation and ethnic symbolism play an important and legitimate role; designs should attempt to work with these priorities, by, for example, developing acceptable substitutes for high fat ingredients in respected recipes.

● Interventions should not assume belief in the health value of slimness, and should be prepared to elicit, and engage constructively with, beliefs in the healthiness of large body size, which have their parallels in, for example, obstetric advice.

Conditions possibly related to vegetarianism

● The aim should be to engage in dialogue with relevant beliefs, since ignorance of the patient's rationale is likely to result in neglect of the advice.

● At present the balance of evidence seems to favour interventions to promote use of supplements rather than dietary change, as being more effective in improving vitamin D status (see 'Rickets and osteomalacia' in Section 2 above).

Infant health and infant feeding practices

● Improve the training in nutrition of midwives and health visitors.

● Improve midwives' and health visitors' understanding of South Asian diet and cultural practices. Given the perceived overall lack of nutritional knowledge of midwives, those working in areas in which South Asians are well represented should be targeted initially.

● Encourage attendance at baby clinics through community-based initiatives.

● Promote and support good infant feeding practice through establishment of mothers' groups in women's centres.

● Encourage ways of incorporating positive 'traditional' values and knowledge of breast-feeding.

Research priorities, including appropriate research questions

General health

We noted at the beginning of Section 4 that the benefit of suggested possible interventions to improve the general health of the South Asian community, rather than the specific conditions below, are hard to assess for lack of relevant research. A good deal of descriptive background needs to be filled in along the following lines:

1. Studies of food purchasing practices (particularly of the elderly with low incomes) are required to determine where South Asians shop and the reasons for their choice of shop.

2. An exploration is needed, in collaboration with other relevant government departments, in low income areas, of ways in which cheaper foods can be made available without contributing to the economic difficulties of South Asian shopkeepers, but rather by harnessing their enterprise to create both food supplies and jobs in such areas.

3. Research on the use of fast-food outlets, especially by children and young people, is needed. Qualitative studies, or qualitative elements within surveys, would identify reasons for their use, for example because of the type of food they provide or because they serve as social meeting places, or for a combination of reasons.

4. Dietary surveys are needed, preferably with measures of nutritional status:

- to judge the extent of the retention of traditional food patterns and the implications of retention or rejection for health in migrant and British-born South Asians

- in workplaces and in schools with substantial proportions of South Asians to determine the range, quality, cultural appropriateness and uptake of South Asian foods supplied institutionally.

Coronary heart disease and control of obesity

- Randomised controlled trials (RCTs) are needed of interventions to reduce central obesity in individuals at risk, by means of diet and exercise, using the suggestions for enhancement of design gathered in the previous section.

- In addition, trials of community interventions are needed, which will probably need to be kept separate from the RCTs above to avoid contamination of control groups. Again suggestions for enhancement of design have been collected in the previous section. Multi-centre before/after designs using differing packages of interventions and publicity will probably be the most economical and informative, provided centres chosen are not those whose South Asian communities have extensive links and diffusion of information to one another.

- Further research is required to determine attitudes to large body size in South Asians, from both health and other social points of view, both in migrants and those born in Britain.

Other social encouragements in reducing fat intake (for example fasts) and obstacles (for example celebratory occasions) also need to be identified, using qualitative methods to explore the context, and also to devise possible means of adapting interventions to these features.

Conditions possibly related to vegetarianism

There seems to have been little or no monitoring of use of vitamin D and iron supplements with associated outcomes among South Asians in recent years (for example Thomas and Avery (1997) show use only); simple projects to link basic data would help to check whether problems have been eliminated or are merely dormant.

Randomised controlled trials are needed of selective interventions to make vitamin D and iron supplements available to those, often women, at risk of deficiency in these respects, using the suggestions for enhancement of design made in the previous section.

Infant health and infant feeding practices

Studies of Sikh and Hindu infant feeding practices could make use of the wide range of incomes found in these groups to differentiate between socioeconomic and cultural influences.

Qualitative studies are needed to determine reasons for observed feeding practices, comparing areas with differing percentages breast-feeding.

A survey is needed of hospital recommendations regarding feeding practices and the degree of support for South Asian mothers, especially in making suitable arrangements to encourage feeding soon after birth.

3. African-Caribbeans

1. African-Caribbeans in context

Geographical distribution, economic situation and income

The African-Caribbean population is the third largest minority ethnic group in Britain with a little under half a million people defined as Black Caribbean in the 1991 Census (Office of Population Censuses and Surveys (OPCS), 1994), representing 0.9% of the total population of Great Britain. This is likely to be an underestimate as many young African-Caribbean people are thought not to have registered because of liability to 'poll tax' at that time. Neither does the figure include a little over 58 000 in the 'Black – Other' category who described themselves as British (Peach, 1996, p. 3) who may be of Caribbean origin. Of the Black Caribbean population resident in Great Britain in 1991, 54% are British born and 45% were born in the English-speaking Caribbean. Of the latter group, the majority were born in Jamaica (59%), other Independent States (18%), Barbados (9%) and Trinidad and Tobago (4%).

Geographical distribution

Most African-Caribbeans are still resident in the initial areas of settlement where there was a high demand for labour such as London, the West and East Midlands and the North West. The majority (66%) are resident in London, 16% in the West Midlands, 4.8% in the East Midlands and 4.3% in the North West.

Economic situation

Like Pakistanis and Bangladeshis in Great Britain, African-Caribbeans consistently occupy lower-level jobs and experience higher rates of unemployment than whites (Jones, 1993) (Table 9). Table 10 provides data of social class of Black Caribbean men and women aged 16 and over. Only 2.4% of Black Caribbean men and 1% of Black Caribbean women were in social class 1 (professional occupations) compared to 6.7% of the white men and 1.7% of white women, with fewer Black Caribbean men (14.2% v. 27.6%) but more Black Caribbean women (30.3 v. 25.9) in social class 2 (managerial and technical positions) compared to white. Unemployment rates were also higher among Black Caribbean men (23.8%) and women (13.5%) compared to white men (10.7%) and women (6.3%) aged 16 and over.

Income

Average full-time hourly rates for 'Black' men and women are £6.88, compared to £7.73 for Whites (Church and Summerfield, 1996).

Housing tenure

A little under half of Black Caribbeans live in owner-occupied housing, compared to two-thirds of Whites. The three Black ethnic groups in the UK are considerably more likely than white people to live in rented accommodation and, in this category, Black Caribbeans are most likely to live in public sector property as opposed to private rented accommodation (Owen, 1994b).

Age and gender structure, family composition

Black Caribbeans are older generally than the Black African and 'Black – Other' groups, but younger than whites. The greatest number of Black Caribbeans are aged between 25 and 44 (29.6% male, 35.6% female). While the number of Black Caribbean men (6.5%) and women (9.3%) of pensionable age is considerably smaller than the white majority (13.9% males, 24.8% females), a considerable proportion of Black Caribbeans is approaching retirement (26.2% male, 19.2% female). Table 3 details marital status and family composition.

Nutritional issues

There is very little information available on the diet, food habits or nutritional intake of the African-Caribbean population living in the UK, whether through ignorance that this group may differ in dietary practice from the ethnic majority (Ahmad, 1995), or through an assumption that their practice should become assimilated (Douglas, 1987). Food portion sizes and nutrient composition values of traditional West Indian dishes are also lacking (Sharma, Cade and Cruickshank, 1993). Results of the few studies that have examined the diets of the African-Caribbean population living in the UK are described below.

In the largest study to date, food and nutrient intake of 210 randomly selected subjects (85 men, 125 women) thought to be representative of the African-Caribbean community in inner Manchester was assessed using a food frequency questionnaire (FFQ) developed specifically for this population. The questionnaire assessed usual food habits as well as nutrient intake during the previous 12 months and contained 108 food items including both traditional West Indian and European foods (Sharma, Cade and Cruickshank, 1993; Sharma *et al.*, 1996). The composition of the diet of this study population is compared in Table 4 with results for those aged 50–64 years in the national survey of Gregory *et al.* (1990) obtained by 7 days' weighed intake, which varied little by age.

There was little difference in the composition of the diets of African-Caribbean men and women, the greatest being that the men consumed

2.3% more of their total energy as alcohol. However, the composition of the diets of the African-Caribbean population is different from that of the mainly White national population with a greater percentage of energy provided by carbohydrate and a lower percentage provided by fat. These results for the women are similar to those obtained in North West London where a small study using 5-day weighed intakes assessed the composition of the diets of 23 African-Caribbean and 37 White (provenly non-diabetic) women (Thompson and Cruickshank, 1990 and Cruickshank and Thompson, unpublished). The diets of the African-Caribbean women were similarly lower in fat and higher in carbohydrate than those of the White women (fat AfC 35.8% v. White 38.1%; carbohydrate AfC 45.2% v. White 43.4%).

Miller *et al.* (1988) carried out a 5-day weighed intake study to examine dietary and other characteristics relevant to CHD in men aged 45–54 years of Indian, West Indian (mainly from Jamaica) and European descent sampled from a general practice. Again the diets of this small African-Caribbean group ($n = 11$) were lower in fat than the diets of the White population (fat AfC 32.6% v. White 38.2%). However, in contrast to the Manchester study, alcohol intake was greater in the 11 West Indian compared with the 20 White men (AfC 6.8% v. 3.5% White). Dowler and Calvert (1995) examined the diets of African-Caribbean, African and White lone parents using 3 days' weighed records and a food frequency questionnaire. Those from Afro-Caribbean or Black British households had a lower percentage energy provided by fat and in particular saturated fat (fat AfC 36.3% v. White 38.9%; saturated fat AfC 10.2% v. White 14.2%). Parents who were Black had more total variety, more fish, vegetables, cereal and fruit variety than White parents, as did their children, and better iron intakes. Eating a typical Afro-Caribbean diet was strongly associated with a high positive healthy dietary score.

Lip *et al.* (1995) assessed the amount of fat contained in food purchases in an average week in three groups of pregnant women (African-Caribbeans, Asians and Whites) attending Dudley Road Hospital, Birmingham. They found that the African-Caribbean group had the lowest median weekly fat in purchased foods. This study looked only at fat purchases and not consumption using a somewhat crude adjustment for household size. No allowance was made for use of fat, and purchases eaten outside the home were not included. However, as with previous individual studies, the results were clearly consistent with lower fat food purchasing and hence lower fat intake.

These data suggest that *on average*, this population is already meeting the COMA (Department of Health, 1994a, p. 2) recommendation of 'a reduction in the average contribution of total fat to dietary energy in the population to about 35%'; the mean percentage energy provided by fat in

Manchester was 32%. COMA also recommended that the 'proportion of dietary energy derived from carbohydrates should increase to approximately 50 per cent'; the mean percentage energy provided by carbohydrate in Manchester African-Caribbeans was over 50%. However, because these are statements about *averages*, many individuals will be eating more dietary fat than is recommended.

The two nutrition-related conditions that have become major contributors to morbidity and mortality for British African-Caribbeans are diabetes and hypertension (Cruickshank, 1989; Cooper *et al.*, 1997; Marmot, Adelstein and Bulusi, 1984; Balarajan, 1995; Forrest, Jackson and Yudkin, 1986; McKeigue, Miller and Marmot, 1991; Cruickshank *et al.*, 1991; Chaturvedi, McKeigue and Marmot, 1993; Cruickshank, Riste and Amica, 1994; Odugbesan *et al.*, 1989; two earlier occupational studies with variant results, Meade, Brozovic and Chakraborti, 1978 and Cruickshank *et al.*, 1985). Some of these surveys combined African-Caribbeans with small numbers of directly African origin except Cruickshank *et al.*, but hypertension prevalence is little different and high at over 30%.

Community diabetes prevalence among African-Caribbeans over 40 years of age is 17% (95% confidence interval 16–18%) from the four population studies (Forest, Jackson and Yudkin, 1986; McKeigue, Shah and Marmot, 1991; Cruickshank *et al.*, 1991; Chaturvedi, McKeigue and Marmot, 1993), with recent work in Manchester (Riste, 1997; Mbanya *et al.*, in press) no different, and similar to current estimates in Jamaica (Morrison and Richards, 1985; Alleyne *et al.*, 1989; Mbanya *et al.*, in press). As in any population, both conditions are strongly related to preceding and current BMI (see above and Cruickshank *et al.*, 1985; Cruickshank and Alleyne, 1987; Khaw and Marmot, 1983; Di Giovanni *et al.*, 1983). These conditions are accompanied by lower risk of IHD which appears to persist even in people with diabetes at generally higher IHD risk (Chaturvedi and Fuller, 1996; Chaturvedi *et al.*, 1996), although selective return migration may be an issue. Cruickshank (1993) has reviewed issues of weight and obesity in relation to blood pressure and diabetes.

Besides body mass, a number of non-dietary influences may be involved in these differences, and it is not clear whether they are also due to differences in risk factors apart from, or secondary to, body mass, for instance blood lipids and coagulation, which are both subject to dietary influence (Miller *et al.*, 1988; Lane *et al.*, 1993). Manolio and colleagues (1995) reviewed these possibilities in the US setting. However, lifestyle factors, most especially obesity and energy imbalance, are likely to explain much if not most of the high prevalence (King and Dowd, 1990).

All studies have shown the BMI of African-Caribbean women particularly, and to some degree men, to be consistently greater than that of White women and men (Meade, Brozovic and Chakaborti, 1978; Cruickshank *et al.*, 1985, 1991; McKeigue, Shah and Marmot, 1991; Chaturvedi, McKeigue and Marmot, 1993; Cruickshank *et al.*, 1996, subsampled by Sharma, 1996). In the United States a higher prevalence of obesity has also been observed among Black women (Kumanyika, 1995; McNabb, Quinn and Rosing, 1993; Kanders *et al.*, 1994; Melnyk and Weinstein, 1994; Burke *et al.*, 1992).

Physical activity is an essential component of energy balance. A recent study suggests lower levels of activity in African-Caribbeans than in the UK population as a whole (Rudat, 1994, p. 53). Rates of physical activity were minimal in both African-Caribbean and White subjects in Manchester (Riste, 1997).

2. Studies specifically concerned with food choice

Specific information is limited, but it is likely that some of the barriers with which African-Caribbeans are confronted will correspond to those met by South Asians, because of shared experience as ethnic minorities in Great Britain.

Access: economic, material and structural barriers and opportunities

Barriers and opportunities presented by social class, income or access to food retail outlets

The traditional African-Caribbean diet tends to be based on a staple of rice or starchy roots, fruits or tubers such as yam, cassava and sweet potato usually accompanying a meat (for example curried mutton) or fish dish (for example red snapper, escovitch) (Douglas, 1987; Sharma *et al.*, 1996). Most of these vegetables are purchased from local markets or stores specialising in African-Caribbean foods in areas where there is a sizable African-Caribbean population. A description of the traditional foods is given in Table 8. These traditional foods, being imported, are more expensive than the European equivalent; for example in 1993 one pound of sweet potato cost 77p compared to one pound of 'Irish' potatoes costing just 14p. Despite this, the majority of African-Caribbean people sampled in Manchester were choosing to buy these imported foods (Sharma, 1996).

In the study of lone parents which included 65 Black Caribbean/Black British/Black African lone parents (Dowler and Calvert, 1995), total and adjusted household income (adjusting for household size and composition) were not significantly different in Black households compared to Whites and there was no significant difference in the mean estimated amount spent on food each week (adjusted). Black parents worried more than White about running out of money for food although there were no differences in material circumstances, budgeting strategies, food aims or shopping practices. Black parents were also more likely to live in larger households although the associations were not strong.

Overall, however, African-Caribbeans are economically disadvantaged in comparison to the ethnic majority and to Indians. Since income influences not only the variety and quality of food which can be purchased but also the type and location of food outlets chosen, some African-Caribbeans may be constrained in these respects.

Older and elderly members of ethnic minorities may be particularly likely to be confronted by barriers to nutritional health such as low income. Although 83 per cent of African-Caribbeans surveyed in Birmingham received a state pension (compared to 94 per cent of 'Europeans' and only 46 per cent of 'Asians'), 42 per cent of African-Caribbeans had a weekly income of less than £20 compared to 17 per cent of Europeans and 38 per cent of Asians (Bhalla and Blakemore, 1981). These data are now rather old, but are supported by the findings of a small inter-regional study that found a quarter of older 'Caribbeans' would like 'additional financial help' (Askham, Henshaw and Tarpey, 1995, p. 92).

Barriers and opportunities presented by institutional menus
Data are available concerning the use of social services by the elderly. Only 2 per cent of 179 African-Caribbeans surveyed in Birmingham received Meals-on-Wheels, although the proportion of ethnic majority elderly receiving them was also small (6 per cent) (Bhalla and Blakemore, 1981). Askham, Henshaw and Tarpey (1995) report 2 per cent of 83 African-Caribbeans ever having used this service, compared to 2 per cent of 89 South Asians, but a slightly greater percentage of the former (23%) had used a lunch club than the latter (18%). Such under-usage could represent a barrier to nutritional health, particularly if the elderly are at all incapacitated or live alone, and are thus unable or not motivated to cook for themselves; a third of African-Caribbeans in Askham's survey lived alone. An open question asked those not currently receiving social services which they would like to have or would have need of in the future; 49% of African-Caribbeans mentioned domestic help. A particularly illuminating finding of this survey is that, while older and elderly African-Caribbeans said that a special diet would be important for them in hospital, only 39 per cent expressed this view, considerably fewer than the 93 per cent of South Asians who did so. Further, 'ethnic issues' were much less of an issue for African-Caribbeans than for South Asians with regard to suggestions for improvements in the services (p. 93). Issues of food provision by social services and health authorities and its appropriateness are discussed in

detail in the review of South Asians.

Barriers and opportunities in access to food information

Chapter 2 noted the frequent reference in the literature to issues of information, with lack of appropriate knowledge on the part of health professionals and South Asians, differences in 'traditional' and biomedical opinion, and problems with communicating information being highlighted. These are shared in some respects by African-Caribbeans. For example, a study of infant feeding practices of 102 mothers (aged 18–41 years) in Birmingham (Kemm, Douglas and Sylvester, 1986; Douglas, 1989) (see below) concluded there is a need for health professionals to be more aware of African-Caribbean infant feeding practices. Most women acknowledged information and advice regarding the infant feeding practices from their mothers or mother-in-laws rather than from doctors, health visitors or midwives, but said they would have liked to have had more information on infant feeding and weaning (Douglas, 1989).

Bhalla and Blakemore (1981) found that 80% of African-Caribbeans they surveyed knew of the existence of Meals-on-Wheels, and 36 per cent knew of lunch clubs; this is in marked contrast to the small number of South Asians who were aware of these facilities.

Potrykus (1991), outlined the health needs of the African-Caribbean population in Wandsworth and concluded that there was inadequate provision for ethnic minorities and particularly African-Caribbeans. She concluded that there was a failure to recognise and cater for the special needs of this significant section of the community. For example, there were no Look-after-your-heart groups aimed at this community and no centre available to provide nutritional support or advice.

Culture and food choice
Barriers and opportunities presented by dietary affiliation and place of birth

The majority of people still eat cooked dishes prepared in the home, many dishes taking up to 3 hours to prepare. However, fast-foods such as patties, dumplings and saltfish fritters are usually available from take-aways as are some of the main meal dishes such as rice and peas with mutton curry. Desserts are seldom eaten as part of a meal (Carlson, Kipps and Thompson, 1984).

A study carried out in Manchester presents the results for the African-Caribbean population, dividing the sample into those people eating a traditional diet (defined as consuming traditional West Indian foods 5–7 days each week) and non-traditional eaters (those eating West Indian foods 0–4 days each week) (Sharma, 1996). This was defined from the subject's response to the question 'On average how many days each week would you consume traditional West Indian foods?' Foods defined as traditional are shown in Table 9, included because they are commonly eaten in Jamaica and some of the other Caribbean islands. Note that some foods share the same name as European foods but the method of preparation or ingredients used are different and hence so is the nutritional composition.

Nutrient intake results were also examined for people born in the Caribbean compared to those born in England (Sharma, 1996). Those born in England were younger and had a lower BMI than subjects born in the Caribbean. Consumption of West Indian foods was more frequent in those born in the Caribbean although English-born subjects consumed traditional foods almost 3 days per week. Again, there was little difference in macronutrient contribution to energy between Caribbean-born men and women. This was lower in fat, higher in carbohydrate and lower in alcohol than the diets of those born in England.

Barriers and opportunities presented by patterns of eating according to gender, age and family processes (including child-rearing practices)

In the Manchester study described above, the composition of the diets of those following a traditional diet was compared to those following a more European-type diet. Those men eating a traditional diet had significantly more energy provided by carbohydrate and less energy provided by fat. Thus eating a 'traditional' diet is a continuing opportunity for African-Caribbean men to achieve good nutritional health. There was no significant difference for women in the composition of traditional and non-traditional diets.

Those men and women following a traditional diet were older (men on average by 6 years and women by 5 years) than those following a non-traditional diet. In total 90% of men and 89% of women eating a traditional diet were born in the Caribbean, compared to 79% of men and 70% of women eating a non-traditional diet (Sharma, 1996).

Infant feeding methods of 102 mothers (aged 18–41 years) were examined as part of the study of African-Caribbean dietary practices in Birmingham (Kemm, Douglas and Sylvester, 1986; Douglas, 1989). The majority of mothers (91%) initiated breast-feeding but this fell, by 8 weeks, to 78%, and by 3 months to 34%, corresponding to the practice of a short period of breast-feeding in the Caribbean, i.e. 3 or 4 months but often less than 1 month (Caribbean Food and Nutrition Institute, 1984, cited in Douglas, 1989). The greatest predictor of breast-feeding for more than 1 month in Birmingham was whether subjects owned their homes. In the Caribbean, semi-solid food was found to be introduced at less than 1 month; this was mainly home-made porridge (cornmeal and banana) as well as commercial products in later months. Traditional weaning practices were followed in African-Caribbean households in Birmingham, but some British infant feeding patterns were adopted (Douglas, 1989).

Also in Birmingham, Griffiths (1983) reported very low levels of breast-feeding in 'West Indian' women who all originated from Jamaica. Early discontinuation of breast-feeding was attributed to the desire and, often, the necessity to work by West Indian women. Solid food was introduced on average at a little under 6 months, later than in most 'English' families (p. 396) and also later than the Caribbean practice, but earlier than Indian and especially Pakistani women. Foods used for weaning were not documented in this study.

Barriers and opportunities presented by other beliefs, values, knowledge, norms and attitudes

As in most other communities, British African-Caribbeans hold many beliefs about food; some are traditional from the Caribbean while others are because of the influences of advertising. For instance, many believe that the white variety of the cho cho relieves high blood pressure (Douglas, 1987) and that many varieties of bush teas have health-giving properties.

Morgan (1995) found that in a study of 30 African-Caribbean people with hypertension, 17 used herbal remedies, generally bush or bitter teas made of dried herbs such as cerosee. These were believed to purify the blood and cleanse the system. This is similar to practices in Jamaica, for instance of choice and usage of bush tea among people with diabetes (Alleyne *et al.*, 1989).

A common idea found during fieldwork in Manchester was that high calorie milk-based drinks were health-giving and most people consumed these at least once per week (Sharma, 1996). Since over 70% of the population were overweight this additional intake of energy was unnecessary. Tonics were also considered as health-giving and when the contents of a commonly cited 'pick-me-up' was examined, it was found to be 14% alcohol but it was still not considered an alcoholic beverage. Douglas (1987) discusses how some foods may be seen as 'super foods', having great healing powers, for example Irish Moss, linseed and home-made tonics. While these beliefs do not present barriers or opportunities in themselves, they could offer an opportunity as part of a weight control programme. Another belief or food custom is to serve a large portion of food, especially to guests, and to eat such a portion is important as signifying a healthy appetite. This may have implications for the high prevalence of obesity.

Higher parity rates, lower rates of breast-feeding and a more inactive lifestyle have been suggested as possible contributing factors to overweight in Black American populations (Burke *et al.*, 1992). American literature has been used to illustrate some cultural differences in attitudes towards obesity, as no work on this topic among African-Caribbeans in the UK has been found. Kumanyika and colleagues (1993) carried out a study to determine attitudinal and behavioural factors that might contribute to influences on weight problems among 500 Black women who were staff of a clinic ($n = 261$) or clinic attendees ($n = 239$). Of particular interest were the culturally-determined, 'permissive' attitudes toward obesity. The mean BMI was 26.9 kg/m^2 , ranging from 15.1 to 60.4 kg/m^2. Only 36% of severely overweight women (BMI > 32.3) to whom the question was applied, reported that their husband or boyfriend thought they were very overweight, implying that men were tolerant of obesity in their partners. The findings of this study are consistent with some others but in Allison and colleagues' work (1993; 1995) comparing men's views of desirable female body shapes, African-American and Hispanic men were *not* found to prefer overweight women. However, they also found African-American *women's* views of themselves to be tolerant of being overweight and others suggest that Black women may be less preoccupied with dieting and have somewhat more tolerant attitudes towards obesity than White women (Kanders *et al.*, 1994; Melnyk and Weinstein, 1994).

The acceptability of a high BMI in women may be a barrier to changing dietary habits, and in some sense may also be regarded as a protective social mechanism in a relatively alien environment. However, if the community were to become more aware of the beneficial effects of restricting weight gain as well as weight loss for the prevention of diabetes and hypertension, this barrier might be overcome.

The British African-Caribbean community, as most recently found in Manchester, are keenly aware of the high prevalence rates of non-insulin dependent diabetes (NIDDM) and high blood pressure (HBP) among the community. This can be deduced from the rates of known:unknown diabetes in testing in a community sample; for African-Caribbeans, the ratio is 2 known to 1 unknown, whereas in the low-prevalence White populations, it is about 1:1 (Cruickshank *et al.*, 1991; Chaturvedi, McKeigue and Marmot, 1993). In Manchester, where over 300 homes were visited, the majority of people asked how they could protect themselves against these conditions experienced by older family and friends and many asked what dietary modifications were necessary (Sharma, 1996).

Interventions with African-Caribbeans

A primary care initiative has been set up in Tower Hamlets, East London. The Healthy Eastenders Project (Falshaw, 1993) involves the staff of 17 GP practices working to common protocols with a view to prevention of cardiovascular and specific cancers. They have undertaken training to take diet histories and to give dietary advice appropriate to African-Caribbean as well as Bangladeshi and Chinese patients. Working with local communities they have produced health education material to replace existing inappropriate information which made little reference to cardiovascular disease. No evaluation of this intervention accompanied the description of this intervention.

In their review of mortality and morbidity from cardiovascular disease and stroke in African-Caribbeans in Great Britain, McKeigue and Chaturvedi (1996, p. 81) note that weight reduction seems to be 'the intervention of choice' to reduce blood pressure in this group. They point out, however, that while early studies in America suggested the lifestyles of blacks and whites could be modified, a more recent study of weight change associated with interventions (Kumanyika *et al.*, 1991) noted that African-Americans' weight loss was consistently less than that of whites. They underline the lack of understanding of dietary composition and of cultural beliefs and values of African-Caribbeans in Great Britain, and point out that communities do not necessarily share dietary preferences.

The central potential role of reducing dietary salt intake in the diet of the African-Caribbean community to help reduce blood pressure has not been adequately examined. Clearly this would involve the three main levels at which intake is determined – in types of (preserved) foods, in cooking and at the table, while maintaining or increasing potassium sources which may also be help blood pressure reduction (Cappuccio *et al.*, 1991).

3. Looking to the future

Socioeconomic trends in African-Caribbeans and inter-generational changes

The studies in Manchester (Sharma, 1996) and in Birmingham (Kemm, Douglas and Sylvester, 1986) showed that the African-Caribbean population were purchasing more expensive imported Caribbean foods and thus, because of lower incomes, a larger proportion was spent on food. The high cost of these traditional foods is likely to be an increasing problem for the growing elderly population. Possibly however, this provides commercial opportunities for local growing in Britain of some of these foods, perhaps under greenhousing. This may particularly suit vegetables including Caribbean pumpkin, egg plants (aubergine) and the 'peas' (red kidney beans) of 'rice and peas' (the Jamaican-origin dish) and black-eye beans for the 'peas and rice' dish of the eastern Caribbean. Such entrepreneurship could be successfully encouraged among the Caribbean-origin community particularly if specifically targeted small grant schemes were available.

Trends in marketing and retailing and the likely impact upon patterns of food choice

No material on these topics peculiar to ethnic minorities was found. The review of barriers and opportunities encountered by South Asians described the impact which changes in retailing, particularly the development of the supermarket system and the decline of small specialist shops, could have upon food choice, and these are likely to affect African-Caribbeans similarly.

4. Research and intervention priorities

Practical suggestions on potential interventions

While the greatest identified barrier to change in the African-Caribbean community is the high prevalence and possible acceptability of obesity, the greatest facilitating factors are:

1. The generally excellent quality of the diet, a highly positive message which needs to be widely employed, while also promoting efforts to reduce the quantity of this intake and/or to increase levels of physical activity.

2. The interest within this community in reducing the incidence of both diabetes and high blood pressure. This can be coupled with the still encouraging position in relation to coronary heart disease which among African-Caribbeans is again already at or below the target levels set in *The health of the nation* for the general population (giving weight to the dietary fat–CHD hypothesis). That position is already showing signs of negative shift for younger African-Caribbeans. Practical suggestions that require relatively small changes to be made to the diet should be encouraged and these should be appropriate to the foods being eaten by this community.

Simple suggestions to reduce obesity, sugar and sodium intake which could form the contents of a health education package that should be formally testable in applied research are described below.

A. Practical points to help weight control and reduction include:

- roast meat and chicken without browning first
- once the fish/meat has been fried dispose of the oil rather than using it as the base for the next stage of cooking
- drink fruit juice or low calorie squash rather than Nutriment/ Nourishment or punch or make equivalents of these drinks with skimmed milk and less sugar; persuading the manufacturers to help is another approach
- try to eat less take-away snack foods such as fried dumplings and patties

- reduce serving size of starchy foods such as yam, sweet potato, plantain and rice
- boil plantains rather than frying
- cut down on alcohol (men)
- try to increase physical activity.

B. Efforts to reduce sugar include:

- reduce what is added to tea/coffee and on cereal
- cut down on Nutriment/Nourishment drinks
- reduce the amount of condensed milk, use ordinary or semi-skimmed milk
- use an unsweetened fruit juice and low sugar squash/syrup
- choose tinned fruit in fruit juice rather than syrup.

C. Efforts to reduce salt intake include:

- aim to use fresh fish more often than salt fish but if the latter, which is becoming scarcer, soak the salt fish overnight in large volumes of water, changing that water at least twice and boiling in fresh water
- cut down on snack foods particularly nuts and crisps
- when marinating and seasoning meat, fish or chicken, use more lemon juice or fresh herbs to flavour so the amount of added salt can be reduced
- try to use less salt/sodium based additives such as MSG and all-purpose seasoning
- use take-away foods such as fried dumplings, salt fish fritters and beef patties as occasional, rather than frequent, foods
- reduce or stop the amount of salt added to cooked dishes including rice and food at table.

Enhancing the design of future dietary intervention strategies

The design of intervention studies should be decided upon only after informed discussion and consultation with members of the community to identify both the mode of communication thought to be most useful with this population and to determine what dietary modifications are believed to be worthwhile and feasible. This could be undertaken by meeting in community places to explain how increased rates of obesity are associated with diabetes and hypertension and, through the involvement of community members, by asking for and employing people's suggestions on these and other issues that may not be perceived to be scientifically relevant but without which people's will to participate will be minimal. 'A key message from US interventions studies is that interventions must be culturally appropriate, and targets achievable for those with limited resources' (McKeigue and Chaturvedi, 1996, p. 82).

One method to establish the preferred means of communication would be using small focus group discussions. Following on from this, appropriate and culturally acceptable good quality materials, made or written with the full involvement of the community such as videos, written materials and audiotapes need to be developed. Some of these are being developed but will need amending in the light of community experience and response.

Once such initiatives are undertaken and accepted, not only is there a likely receptive audience but also one that is relatively easy to target as most members of the community meet regularly in local churches, luncheon clubs, youth centres, day clubs, etc. These meeting places are used by people of all ages. Ethnic-specific media, including radio and newspapers such as *The Voice* and many others, may well be interested in taking up these issues.

There is clearly increasing awareness in the African-Caribbean population of the importance of diet in the prevention of disease and maintenance of good health. Some of the data in this review should help the development of clear guidelines for dietary information specific to this group not yet available.

Research priorities, including appropriate research questions

1. Continuing research needs to assess dietary preferences of this population in other representative samples apart from Manchester; other studies to date have been on small numbers or among specific sub-groups such as lone parents. The availability of a food frequency questionnaire designed to assess the diets of this population could allow this instrument to be modified and used elsewhere in the UK with relatively little extra work. Others, also calibrated against different methods of nutritional assessment, may need to to be developed.

2. Intervention trials (probably multicentre) on modification of salt intake and its relation to high blood pressure among African-Caribbeans. Stratifying so that adequate numbers of younger people are recruited would seem appropriate.

3. Methods:

Research is needed to develop methods which might be used among this population group:

(a) to help maintain the *quality* of traditional elements of the African-Caribbean diet and to promote pride in this as an example that already meets national dietary targets;

(b) to combine this with some focus on reducing dietary *quantity* in relation to weight control and reduction across the community.

4. Research is need in this population group to develop methods of promoting appropriate physical activity to help energy balance patterns that reduce obesity, particularly in younger people.

Continuing research issues include:

● Community:

More generalisable data are required on the following:

1. Nutritional patterns and food choices, particularly among non-Jamaican origin African-Caribbean adults, and African-Caribbean schoolchildren in general.

2. Household attitudes to food choices and data on who does the buying and cooking (knowing, not surmising or assuming).

3. Attitudes to obesity; interrelations with *physical activity* promotion.

4. Marketing/retailing responsiveness.

5. Attitudes of health professionals – stereotyping.

6. Effective methods of intervention – in schoolchildren and adolescents, in women before having children and in adults generally.

● Laboratory field work:

More research is needed in the following areas:

1. Effective methods of measuring physical activity in African-Caribbeans compared with other groups.

2. Relationships of nutritional intakes to total energy expenditure.

3. How energy expenditure relates to both longer-term risk of, as well as newly detected, high blood pressure and diabetes as the major health outcomes of obesity in this population.

This restricted list reflects virtually no data on interventions of a public health type among African-Caribbeans in Britain. A small pilot is in progress in Manchester among people who are overweight but relatively poor response rates perhaps indicate limitations of targeted rather than community approaches, for instance through churches, youth and older adult groups.

4. The Irish

1. The Irish in context

Irish migration to Britain has been substantial since the 1800s, peaking in the middle of last century (Chance, 1996; Williams, 1992) and again in the 1960s (Owen, 1995). Although the Irish form the largest minority ethnic in Britain (Chance, 1996), until recently they have not been considered as a distinct ethnic group because of the common confusion between ethnicity and race. The Census category 'born in Ireland' acts as a 'surrogate Irish ethnic group', but does not always permit differentiation between migrants from the Republic and from Northern Ireland, and obviously excludes those of Irish descent born in Britain (Chance, 1996, p. 221). Information on the health of groups born in Britain has only recently begun to emerge, using data on country of birth of parents (for example in the ONS Longitudinal Study, but usually only available for parents from the Irish Republic), or data on religion, usually only including descendants of Irish Catholics (for example Abbotts *et al.*, 1997), who have formed 93–5% of the population of the Republic, and 31–4% of the population of Northern Ireland in the period since the partition of Ireland (Currie, Gilbert and Horsley, 1977, pp. 220–2). While intermarriage between Irish-born migrants is relatively low (Caulfield and Bhat, 1981), there is some evidence of high levels of intermarriage among Catholics in areas where they are recruited largely from both Irish migrants and people of Irish descent (Williams, 1993a). Studies of identity and heterogeneity in these British-born groups are beginning to appear (Hickman, 1995), as are studies of mortality and morbidity discussed below.

The 1991 Census recorded 836 934 Irish-born people living in Britain, 71 per cent of whom were born in the Republic (including 'Ireland, part not stated') and 29 per cent in the North (Chance, 1996). The inclusion of British-born people of Irish descent would substantially increase the total, as percentages of Irish-born in nineteenth-century populations were much higher.

Geographical distribution, economic situation and income
Geographical distribution
The geographical distribution of the two Irish birth groups is very different. Those born in the Republic are more strongly concentrated, with over half living in the South East of England, and more than a third

in Greater London. Other major concentrations occur in the metropolitan counties of the West Midlands, Greater Manchester, South and West Yorkshire and Merseyside. In contrast, Northern Irish-born are distributed across Great Britain as a whole, and are especially well represented in Scotland and the North West of England (Owen, 1995; Chance, 1996). At the height of migration from Ireland to Britain in the middle of the last century, the adult populations of Liverpool, Glasgow and Dundee consisted of 29 per cent, 23 per cent and 22 per cent Irish-born respectively; these cities, together with most major urban centres in the north and west, remain focuses of populations of Irish descent (Williams, 1993b).

Economic situation
Employment
Men who have migrated from the Republic and Northern Ireland to Britain are generally over-represented in manual work (8.8% of Irish males are unskilled manual workers) and under-represented in white collar work, although 6.9% are in social class I as opposed to 6.7% of 'white' men. Lower percentages of Irish-born men are in class II (managerial and technical) and class III (skilled non-manual work) than 'white' men. However, higher percentages of Irish-born women are in classes I and II than 'white' women. Otherwise, like men, they are over-represented in class V (unskilled manual) (Chance, 1996). Northern Irish-born men work mainly in service jobs, while almost one-third of those from the Republic are in construction work. Nursing is an important source of employment for women from the North and the Republic (Owen, 1995). Irish-born men are more likely than 'white' but less likely than South Asian men to be self-employed. Table 9 details the economic activity of the Irish-born in Britain.

Unemployment
Unemployment rates for Irish-born men and women are higher than for 'whites' (only marginally higher for women) but lower than South Asians with the exception of Indians (Table 9). However, rates for men and women born in Northern Ireland are lower than for those born in the Republic (Owen, 1995).

Income
Income figures are not available for Irish-born in Britain. The analysis of the 1988–1990 Labour Force Survey (Jones, 1993) does not consider the Irish in Britain as a separate minority ethnic.

Housing tenure
The 1991 Census reports 55% of Irish-born in Britain owning their own property, compared to 67% of 'whites' and 82% of Indians. Twenty-six per cent of Irish were in council housing (or the Scottish equivalent), compared to 21% of all households (Chance, 1996). The percentage of

Irish-born renting from the private sector is comparable to 'minority ethnic groups' but well above the average for 'all white households' (Owen, 1995, p. 9). The Irish are greatly over-represented in the categories which relate to homelessness (hostels, common lodging houses, and sleeping rough), and young Irish appear to be particularly likely to be without permanent accommodation. Irish-born are also over-represented in hospital staff residences, reflecting the high numbers who work in the health-care sector (Chance, 1996).

Age and gender structure, family composition

The Irish-born in Britain are, on average, older than the rest of the population, and those born in the Republic of Ireland have an even older age distribution than those born in the North. Only 6% of males and 5.7% of females born in the North, and 3.3% males and 3.4% females born in the Republic are under the age of 15. For all Irish-born, females are in the majority throughout the age profile and outnumber men most strongly in the oldest groups. However, 13% more men than women between the ages of 44–64 were born in the Republic (Owen, 1995). Details of family composition and marital status are set out in Table 11.

Nutritional issues

Almost nothing addresses the nutritional health of the Irish in Britain; the neglect of 'white' ethnic minorities in the literature has led to the virtual exclusion of the Irish from reviews of health (Ahmad, Sheldon and Stuart, 1996). The profound implications of the lack of nutritional data are made clear by evidence for the health disadvantage of the Irish in Britain (Balarajan, 1996; Balarajan and Bulusu, 1990; Marmot, Adelstein and Bulusi, 1984; Raftery, Jones and Rosato, 1990). This disadvantage includes the British-born (Abbotts *et al.*, 1997); Harding and Balarajan, 1996), and in the past high mortality occurred in British cities with large numbers of Irish despite low levels of mortality in Ireland (Williams, 1994).

In one of the few studies of Irish migrants, dietary variation in three male cohorts was assessed (Kushi *et al.*, 1985). A number of significant differences were found, with men born and living in Ireland having higher energy intakes than their brothers now resident in Boston and than the third cohort of non-related men of Irish descent in Boston. Their intake of animal fats was also greater, and their fibre intake lower than the other two groups. The significantly higher relative weight of migrant compared with non-migrant brothers, coupled with the higher energy intake of the non-migrants, indicates that physical activity was also greater in Ireland than in Boston. Data on these indicators among migrants to Britain would be of value. The evidence that Irish migrants may fare differently from the Irish in Ireland enforces caution, but some clues may nevertheless be available from patterns in Ireland, where conditions are closer to those in Britain than in the case of the other minorities discussed here. In 1992 a National Nutrition Surveillance Centre was set up in University College Galway. The first annual report (Newell, Nolan and Kelleher, 1993), a comprehensive survey of factors influencing nutrition in Ireland, was followed by a short report focusing on morbidity and health status (Friel, Nolan and Kelleher, 1995). In addition, reports of national dietary surveys of the Republic (Irish Nutrition and Dietetic Institute, 1990) and of Northern Ireland (Barker *et al.*, 1989) are available.

The Irish National Nutrition Survey was conducted in 1989 and used seven-day diet histories to obtain data on food and nutrient intakes of 1214 people aged 8 years and older living in the Republic (Irish Nutrition and Dietetic Institute, 1990). The diets of a random sample (616) of the adult population of Northern Ireland were reported in a survey of diet, lifestyle and health in the province, conducted in 1986–87 (Barker *et al.*, 1989). Comparisons here are limited to adult intakes of energy, fat, fibre and iron (Tables 5 and 6), because the Northern Ireland survey did not report vitamin intakes and because of the relevance of these dietary components for the aetiology of common chronic disease.

Energy intakes were generally higher for men and women in the Republic than in Northern Ireland and Great Britain. The Irish staples of bread, potatoes, milk and meat contributed 55% of total energy intake in the Republic, with biscuits, cakes, table sugar and confectionery contributing 18%. In Northern Ireland, the major sources of energy were bread, cereals, potatoes, biscuits, cakes and puddings, contributing 45.9% and 47.8% of energy content of the diet for men and women respectively; women obtained a higher proportion of energy from biscuits, cakes, puddings, fruit, vegetables, nuts and meat products than did men (Barker *et al.*, 1989).

Mean percentage of energy intake (including alcohol) from total fat was lower for men and women in the Republic compared to the North, and to Great Britain (Gregory *et al.*, 1990), and were closer to the COMA recommendation of below 35% of energy intake (including alcohol).

The COMA report supports the view that the term 'dietary fibre' is now obsolete, preferring to recommend a figure (18g/day) for non-starch polysaccharides (NSP) which constitute the major part of 'dietary fibre' (Department of Health, 1991, p. 61). However, fibre intakes rather than NSP are specified in the reports cited here, so are compared to the NACNE recommendation (1983) of 30 g/day (cited in Gregory *et al.*, 1990). Both Irish samples and the British sample fell below this recommendation, with women's intakes considerably lower than men's in all three samples.

Intakes of iron in the Republic were generally greater than in Northern Ireland for men and women, but intakes in both Irish samples were generally lower than in Great Britain for men and women (see also Armstrong, 1989). Overall, iron intakes of men and women aged 50 and over were in excess of the COMA recommendations, but intakes of other women were below them.

Various nutrition-related conditions have been noted in Irish groups in Britain or Ireland:

1. *Reduced stature*. In Clydeside having Catholic parents or being born Catholic is indicative of Irish Catholic descent, and evidence has been examined for these differences by religion and social class in three cohorts aged 18, 38 and 58 (Abbotts *et al.*, 1997). Catholics were shorter than non-Catholics in all cohorts (though this was not a significant difference for the youngest cohort when controlled for social class). Comparison of (limited) Irish and British data shows no evidence of a difference in height, making a genetic explanation unlikely. A relationship exists between body size and poverty which is thought to be mediated by poor dietary intake and infection (Martorell, 1985).

2. *Coronary heart disease*. Standardised mortality rates for CHD of Irish-born living in Britain have been greater than the England and Wales rates at each decennial analysis since 1970–2 (Marmot, Adelstein and Belusu, 1984; Britton, 1990; Balarajan, 1995). The same is true of rates for second-generation Irish (Harding and Balarajan, 1996). The relationship of diet to CHD aetiology in Irish migrants to the USA is supported 'albeit weakly' by the Ireland–Boston Diet–Heart Study (Kushi *et al.*, 1985, p. 811). Mortality rates from CHD in the Republic are high (Shelley *et al.*, 1995) (higher than England and Wales, though lower than Scotland) and for Northern Ireland are the highest in the world (Boreham *et al.*, 1993). The rate of decline in CHD rates in Ireland between 1970 and 1988 is less marked than in other countries, and an increase in CHD morbidity in the Republic is suggested by increased hospital admission rates (Newell, Nolan and Kelleher, 1993; Friel, Nolan and Kelleher, 1995; Shelley *et al.*, 1995). Studies in the Republic and Northern Ireland indict high mean total or saturated fat intakes and low fibre intakes (Gibney, Moloney and Shelley, 1989; Evans *et al.*, 1995; Boreham *et al.*, 1993).

3. *Obesity* (Department of Health, 1991). Higher waist–hip ratios of groups in two cohorts of men and women (38 and 58 years) of Irish descent in comparison to non-Irish have been reported in Glasgow (Abbotts *et al.*, 1997). As previously noted, in the 'Boston brothers' study relative weight was significantly higher in the cohort of migrant brothers living in Boston than in the Irish brothers (Kushi *et al.*, 1985). Tables 7 and 8 compare BMI results of studies in the Republic,

Northern Ireland and Britain, using (for men) the criteria of the Royal College of Physicians of London (1983), but variable age divisions. At age 16–64 mean BMI values for Northern Irish and British men and women were similar due to differing age distributions (Table 8), but the proportion of men with BMI > 25 tended to be greater in Northern Ireland (Table 7) (Barker et al., 1989; Gregory et al., 1990). At age 35–64 mean BMI of Republic males tended to be higher than in Britain and males tended to higher percentages with BMI > 25 (Shelley et al., 1991b). Other studies in Ireland also comment on risks of obesity (Evans et al, 1995; Riddoch et al., 1991; Boreham et al., 1993).

4. Cancer. Standardised mortality rates for stomach and colon cancer of Irish-born migrants to Britain have generally been a little higher than rates for England and Wales (Marmot, Adelstein and Belusu, 1984; Britton, 1990). Cancers of the digestive tract have an established link with diet (Friel, Nolan and Kelleher, 1995) and a high fat, low fibre diet appears to contribute to cancer of the large bowel. Mortality figures indicated 'epidemic' proportions of the disease in Ireland in the 1970s (Habba and Doyle, 1982, p. 439; Habba, Daly and Doyle, 1982), and colon cancer continues to be a major cause of cancer deaths in the 1990s (Newell, Nolan and Kelleher, 1993).

5. Neural tube defects (NTD). Total prevalence in Northern Ireland declined significantly for 1980–1988 but at 33.1 per 10 000 the rate for this period is still high, and for Dublin also, compared with South East England (Wright, 1995). Nutritional status, particularly folate (Smithells, 1996), has been indicated in NTD aetiology, in tandem with genetic susceptibility (Wright, 1995; Gibney and Lee, 1989).

2. Studies specifically concerned with food choice

Access: economic, material and structural barriers and opportunities

This section presents evidence for potential barriers to, and opportunities for, access to food which promotes good nutritional health, taking the data in the sequence of the lifecourse. As described earlier, the greater part of the material by far is concerned with the Irish either in the Republic or in Northern Ireland. It is also clear that the element which unifies the evidence is social class, rather than culture, and the literature does not use religion as a basis for comparison as it does in some South Asian studies.

In the absence of other data, studies in Ireland may be useful in giving a preliminary idea of how food choices of Irish people respond to the constraints of low social class, which, at the gross level usually measured, are of a similar order to class constraints in Britain. Social class background in Ireland may also help to illuminate aspects of the nutritional health of Irish migrants in Britain, as may other structural variations of background in Ireland such as rural versus urban location. However, since these aspects of economic background in Ireland do not offer opportunities for British policy interventions, studies of Irish migrants in Britain, which do have implications for British policy, are treated separately in the latter part of each section.

Barriers and opportunities presented by social class, income or access to food

A review of changes in food availability in the Republic summarised the impact of socioeconomic status upon the nutritional wellbeing of the Irish: '. . . much undernutrition still persists in the poorer sections of the population . . . and . . . the general increased affluence of the population has led to an overconsumption of nutrients' (Robertson and Kevany, 1982). An increase in this polarisation of nutritional status may have occurred in the 1980s, through trends bringing about an increase in the number of households in which no one had paid work but also in the number of households with more than one employed member (Newell, Nolan and Kelleher, 1993).

Socioeconomic group has an impact on infant feeding methods. The preliminary report of a survey in the Republic of Ireland of the distribution of feeding methods at the time of discharge from maternity units showed that feeding method was related to socioeconomic group and to marital status; 55 per cent of women in non-manual classes were breast-feeding, as opposed to 16.5 per cent of non-skilled manual; only 9% of unmarried women were breast-feeding (McSweeney and Kevany, 1982). There was also a 'small but consistent rural–urban gradient' (p. 453) in the numbers breast-feeding, 28% of women breast-feeding in villages/rural areas compared to 36% in cities/suburbs. Statistical significance is not reported.

Part of the Kilkenny Health Project (see below) involved the gathering of baseline data on health-related knowledge, attitudes and behaviour in school attenders between the ages of 11 and 19, in order to evaluate health promotion initiatives aimed at young people in the Republic (O'Reilly and Shelley, 1991). Some of the schools involved in the study had taken part in a structured health education programme for a year, but 55 per cent had not received health education. The amount of health education received related to children's social class and age, with younger children and those in the higher social classes receiving more. Smoking and alcohol consumption increased with age, and exercise decreased with age; these factors are not related to social class, and the relationship of food habits and social class is not reported.

There are social class differences in the consumption of dietary fat (Bolton-Smith *et al.*, 1990). Barker and colleagues (1995) studied attitudes to fat and fibre as they relate to food and nutrient intake and lifestyle and sociocultural factors in Northern Ireland. A significant relationship for women between socioeconomic group and attitude to fibre was reported: those from non-manual and manual households had higher pro-fibre scores than those from unemployed and other (economically inactive) households (p. 654); a higher score reflects an increased perception of fibre as health promoting. However, no social class differences were noted in attitudes to dietary fat. We return to this study in the following section to examine gender differences in attitudes to fat and fibre. In the Irish National Survey the highest intakes of fibre were reported in 'the professional category' and the lowest in 'the unemployed category' (Irish Nutrition and Dietetic Institute, 1990, p. 68).

The Kilkenny Health Project reported differences in the social class distribution of obesity for women but not men; there were significantly fewer obese (BMI > 30) women in the lower professional class (class 2) and more in other non-manual and unskilled manual classes (classes 3 to 6) (Shelley *et al.*, 1991b). In Northern Ireland, a lower percentage of women in non-manual classes were obese compared to manual and unemployed, but a lower percentage of unemployed men than non-manual or manual were obese; these differences were not significant (Barker *et al.*, 1989).

Additional analysis of data from the Northern Ireland survey illustrate the link between income and variety of diet (Barker *et al.*, 1990). A diet featuring pasta, rice, pâtés, cooked meats and shell fish was favoured by non-manual workers, both men and women, in Northern Ireland. Gibney and Lee (1989) surveyed a suburb of Dublin with high unemployment and found low mean daily intakes of certain nutrients in women particularly. Iron, folate and fibre were below the COMA DRVs, and also lower than intakes of women in the Irish National Nutrition Survey (Newell, Nolan and Kelleher, 1993). At national level, drawing definite conclusions about differences in dietary intakes across socioeconomic classes was problematic because of the small numbers in categories, but the data suggest that families of the unemployed had the poorest quality diets (Irish Nutrition and Dietetic Institute, 1990, p. 74).

A study of two supermarkets in contrasting socioeconomic areas in Galway found considerable difference in the range and availability of foods between the two (Dineen, 1991). In Ireland, like Britain, the number of smaller shops is declining with the growth of supermarket chains (Newell, Nolan and Kelleher, 1993). A summary of shopping practices of Irish housewives indicates that attitudes to shopping, as well as income, have an impact on where specific purchases are made (p. 110) and we discuss this further below. Some women never buy own-label goods (particularly coffee and tea) which are cheaper, because they are suspected of being inferior to manufacturers' brands; 'hence there is a conflict between quality and price'.

Tilki's (1994) review of the health and social circumstances of older Irish migrants in Great Britain does not consider food habits, but is pertinent since it highlights the poverty in retirement which many older Irish migrants experience as a consequence of 'persistent low socioeconomic status, intermittent employment history and sporadic pension contributions' (p. 911). While noting the lack of documentary evidence, Tilki suggests that elderly Irish men may be especially disadvantaged. The percentage unmarried is twice the national UK average (Pearson *et al.*, 1991, cited in Tilki, 1994), and 'they are less likely to be domesticated, having moved to 'digs' from the ministrations of mothers and sisters'. The potential combination of poverty, solitary living and shortage of domestic skills could be a considerable barrier to good nutritional health in this section of the Irish migrant population in Great Britain. A further obstacle may be the 'desire to avoid the stereotypical attitudes of health professionals' and the desire of some, including health professionals themselves, to avoid being identified as Irish (p. 913), perhaps because of the stereotyping they encounter.

Culture and food choice

As in the previous section, virtually nothing in the literature is pertinent to culture and food choice as it relates to migrants to Britain, and we rely primarily on Irish studies either from the Republic or from Northern Ireland. We note again the absence of religion as a basis for comparison in the relevant literature, which is in marked contrast to reports of South Asians.

Barriers and opportunities presented by dietary variation according to area of origin

As with South Asians, dietary differences by area of origin suggest the possibility of cultural patterns, but until causal pathways are identified no conclusions can be drawn. Dietary variation and differing food practices are evident in rural as opposed to urban backgrounds. The effect on breast-feeding was noted above. Differences also exist with regard to patterns of food consumption; although the same type of diet was eaten in rural and urban areas, proportionately more potatoes and milk, less orange juice and fewer chips were taken in rural areas. Higher potato consumption meant the proportion of energy derived from carbohydrates was higher, and from fat lower, in rural areas (Irish Nutrition and Dietetic Institute, 1990). The Attitudes Study, part of the Kilkenny Health Project, found the idea that eating healthy food is important to be more common in urban respondents than rural (Conroy, 1992, in Newell, Nolan and Kelleher, 1993).

Barriers and opportunities presented by patterns of eating according to gender, age and family processes (including child-rearing practices)

Links have been made between a high fat, low fibre diet and CHD, bowel cancer and obesity. Attitudes to dietary fat and fibre differ by gender in Northern Ireland (Barker, Thompson and McClean, 1995), with women more likely than men to view dietary fat as a threat to health and fibre as more health-promoting. Men with negative attitudes to fat ate smaller amounts of sausages and chips, but greater amounts of beef, butter, cream, cheese and also milk, and various baked goods, suggesting a possible misunderstanding of foods' fat content (p. 655). Women with negative attitudes to fat ate fewer chips and sausages and less butter. Men and women with positive views of fibre ate more through increased consumption of potatoes, vegetables, fruit and wholemeal bread. It appears that fibre-rich foods cause less ambivalence than fat-rich foods, perhaps because of the prestigious nature of the latter (p. 656).

Gender and particularly age are differentiating factors in five groups of consumers in the Republic categorised by their attitudes to food, namely a young group interested in healthy eating but who snack between meals; a further group of young people biased towards fast foods and neither experimental or very concerned with health; a 'low fat' group who are older and more conservative; an older group, mostly male and not concerned with the fat content of food; and the oldest group, men and women with very conservative eating patterns (Anon., 1991, in Newell, Nolan and Kelleher, 1993).

In Northern Ireland, a random sample revealed four dietary patterns which are followed by distinct population groups (Barker *et al.*, 1990). A traditional diet, with a high content of 'staple indigenous foods' (p. 326) and high fat and carbohydrate foods, was associated with older, rural, Roman Catholic males; women were less likely to follow this pattern, but those who did were older. A cosmopolitan diet, including a more 'international' range of foods, and fruit and vegetables, was favoured primarily by women, supporting Charles and Kerr's (1988) finding that women are more amenable than men to dietary change. As 'food providers' they are also more likely to be exposed to messages about the links between food, nutrition and health (Barker *et al.*, 1990, p. 327). The third distinct pattern was based on convenience foods and was followed particularly by younger people, especially men. It suggests the acceptance of 'fast' foods as a dietary practice in Northern Ireland, and the reluctance of men to cook. Finally, although a 'meat and two veg.' diet was favoured by men who drank at least once a week, it was not peculiar to any one sociocultural group, again reinforcing Charles and Kerr's (1988) finding that members of all social classes aspired to this eating pattern (Barker *et al.*, 1990, p. 328).

Aspects of the eating habits of young people in the Republic give cause for concern, particular 'snacking', both in place of 'proper' meals and in addition to them. Crisps, chocolate and Coca Cola are consumed while travelling to school, often in place of breakfast, and an average of six snacks, ranging from cakes and biscuits to beans on toast, pizza and kebabs, may be eaten after the evening meal (Newell, Nolan and Kelleher, 1993). Schoolchildren in County Kilkenny had a high intake of cakes, chocolate, biscuits and crisps, with only 8% of 445 respondents not having eaten one of these snacks on the day prior to completion of the questionnaire. On a more positive note, 74% of pupils reported eating fruit daily, a little over 36% eating fruit more than once a day (O'Reilly and Shelley, 1991), but the evidence indicates that young people in the Republic are generally following a low fibre, high fat diet (Newell, Nolan and Kelleher, 1993). Findings for Northern Ireland schoolchildren are similar, crisps being popular and 15% having no breakfast. However, 65% ate fruit and vegetables at least three times a week (Riddoch et al., 1991).

Turning to family processes, and looking first at infant feeding, a survey of 31 maternity units in the Republic (estimated to cover 90% of births) found 32% of mothers breast-feeding at time of discharge (McSweeney and Kevany, 1982). This finding is comparable to that of Lowry and Lillis (1993), who reported 36% of 877 women who delivered at a single hospital in Galway to be breast-feeding, with up to 10% continuing to do so 5 months postnatally. Convenience and experience were primary considerations in the choice of feeding method.

Meals are influenced by the divergent tastes of family members: Irish men tend to want familiar 'traditional' foods (often simply meat and potatoes, with vegetables being disliked) while children express a preference for burgers, chips, sausages, tinned baked beans and fish fingers and 'are not keen on fish or salads or vegetables (apart from baked beans)' (Anon., 1986, p. 20). In Northern Ireland, family size influenced food choice, with larger families avoiding the 'cosmopolitan' diet described above; 'children's' food such as baked beans and fish fingers were avoided by those following the cosmopolitan diet (Barker et al., 1990, p. 327).

It is reported that 'the Irish housewife' is the family member most likely to be concerned about the health implications of the family diet, but home baking of many goods including bread, cakes and pies continues to be a regular practice of many Irish women, and one which gives an opportunity for creativity, rather than routine family feeding (Anon., 1986). The increased use of convenience foods is also apparently a source of ambivalence since they are quickly prepared but expensive and give rise to the concern that they may not be as beneficial for the family as home prepared food. Given the projected rise in female employment in Ireland (FAS/ESRI employment forecast, cited in Newell, Nolan and Kelleher, 1993, p. 105), their use is unlikely to diminish.

Barriers and opportunities presented by other beliefs, values, knowledge, norms and attitudes

'The basic Irish attitude to food is one that values serving plenty of good plain solid food', rather than that which is elaborate in content or preparation (Anon., 1986, p. 26). Paradoxically, interest in continental cuisines is increasing, and there is a growing number of delicatessen shops in the Republic. Specialist shops are preferred by many for the purchase of fresh meat, fruit vegetables, such foods being considered less fresh in supermarkets, and fresh vegetables are also widely believed to be better than frozen (Anon., 1986; Kearney and Gibney, 1993). There appears to be an element of 'ceremony' in the use of specialist outlets, which is lacking in supermarkets, although the competitive prices of the latter are recognised. Thus there is 'a conflict between quality and price' (Newell, Nolan and Kelleher, 1993, p. 110). Whether a preference for specialist shops presents barriers to, or opportunities for, good nutritional health is unclear, since much depends on the freshness and quality of the food on offer; for example, we have already noted that frozen vegetables from supermarkets and freezer centres may have greater nutrient content than 'fresh' vegetables which lose their nutritional value rapidly after harvesting.

The broadcast media are the primary sources of information about healthy eating in the Republic, although 'doctor/GP' was as frequently mentioned by those aged 65 and over (Kearney and Gibney, 1993). The finding that a particular brand of sunflower margarine was commonly thought to contain fewer calories than butter may indicate the power of commercial advertising to cause confusion in the minds of the public. There is also a tendency for health education messages to target 'bad foods' rather than promoting a generally 'healthy' diet (Newell, Nolan and Kelleher, 1993).

Surveys have revealed a clear connection between food and health in the minds of the Irish in the Republic (Anon., 1986; Anon., 1991, in Newell, Nolan and Kelleher, 1993; Conroy 1992, in Newell, Nolan and Kelleher, 1993; Kearney and Gibney, 1993; McCluskey, 1989). Two-thirds of adults surveyed link longevity with healthy diet, 57% try to eat less fat and 54% try to eat healthier foods (Anon, 1991, in Newell, Nolan and Kelleher, 1993). Even so, some health claims are met with scepticism and some appear to feel that concerns with food choice have gone too far (Anon., 1991, in Newell, Nolan and Kelleher, 1993). It has been suggested that 'long-term dietary change will be influenced in large measure by people's attitude to food and the extent to which they believe it plays a part in illness or disease causation' (Newel, Nolan and Kelleher, 1993, p. 112), but some studies confirm that attitude or knowledge and behaviour are very different things. For example, children taking part in the Kilkenny Health Project were asked a range of questions concerning 'health knowledge' (O'Reilly and Shelley, 1991, p. 42); 73% answered at least two-thirds correctly, but no significant association was found between children's scores and the health behaviours studied, including eating habits. In the North, 75% of boys and 86% girls held the view that eating less fat promoted health, which is taken to indicate their absorption of health education messages (Riddoch et al., 1991). A more detailed dietary survey would indicate whether their understanding and behaviour correlate.

The Attitudes Study, part of the Kilkenny Health Project, found that coronary heart disease (CHD) was not perceived as a major health problem in Ireland; the idea that rather than being simply an acute episode CHD is a chronic condition, and therefore potentially preventable, was unfamiliar. Further there was a lack of belief that longevity could be affected by individual behaviour (Conroy, 1992, in Newell, Nolan and Kelleher, 1993). In view of the severity of CHD in Ireland (Friel, Nolan and Kelleher, 1995) and in Irish migrants (Marmot, Adelstein and Bulusi, 1984) and their descendants in Britain (Harding and Balarajan, 1996) these are important findings.

Interventions with the Irish

Reports of interventions with Irish migrants in Britain are lacking. In their absence, clues about appropriate resource materials and approaches may be obtainable from interventions in Ireland.

The Kilkenny Health Project

This project was set up as a community-based research and demonstration programme for cardiovascular disease prevention in County Kilkenny (South East Ireland), and as a pilot project for future national initiatives. The main goal was to reduce mortality rates from CHD and cerebrovascular disease in 35- to 64-year-olds by 20% over 10 years (Shelley et al., 1991a). The health promotion programme was carried out between 1985 and 1992, and included the review and development of health education materials, community discussion meetings, a nutrition counselling service, health awareness and assessment programmes which were covered by the local media, and special events including a road race. Outcome evaluation was by population surveys in Kilkenny and in the reference country, Offaly (Shelley et al., 1995).

Overall, changes in risk factor levels were similar in County Kilkenny and in Offaly. Serum total cholesterol declined in men (significant for Offaly) and women (both significant), but mean body mass index increased in men (significant in Offaly) and women (both significant). There were significant reductions in the five-year CHD risk in men and women in intervention and control counties (Shelley et al., 1995).

Changes in food choice were observed, with fish, chicken, fruit and vegetables eaten more frequently post-intervention, and a lower percentage of people using butter (Friel, Nolan and Kelleher, 1995; Shelley et al., 1995). It was known that the most effective way of–communicating in Kilkenny was via the national media, but this method was minimised to avoid contaminating the control area; even so, some contamination occurred which may account for the similarity between intervention and control counties (Shelley et al., 1995).

The development and testing of education materials has produced a wide range of materials now available to other community programmes. The project has revealed important attitudinal barriers to behaviour change (Shelley et al., 1995). Resources should be targeted at those with least education and those at increased risk of CHD.

Health at Work
This is a lifestyle intervention in the workplace set up by the Department of Health Promotion, University College, Galway in 1991, as part of a wider initiative, the Europe Against Cancer programme, and is aimed specifically at women. The baseline survey involved 2528 respondents in five sites. Baseline dietary data have been compared to those from Kilkenny (baseline and post-intervention) and the Happy Heart National Survey (Friel, Nolan and Kelleher, 1995). The intervention found that the key to promoting healthy eating is in providing access to healthy options in the canteen and reinforcing the availability of these options through clear, simple and specific messages (Hope and Kelleher, 1995).

3. Looking to the future

Socioeconomic trends in the Irish, and the likely impact upon patterns of food choice
There are considerably greater numbers of Irish-born men and women aged 45–64, especially males born in the Republic (44.5%), in comparison to the rest of the population of Great Britain (Owen, 1995). If they remain in Britain, the percentage of pensionable age will increase dramatically in the coming decades, resulting in considerable numbers whose nutritional and general health may be compromised, since it has been proposed (Tilki, 1994) that older Irish migrants to Britain, especially male, may be at increased risk of economic and social disadvantage. However, this age band covers almost twenty years, and the youngest members (40–49) currently have lower rates of unemployment than those aged 50–59/64; even so, Republic-born males aged 40–49 are considerably more likely than those born in the North and women from both countries to be unemployed (Owen, 1995). Republic-born migrants are also less likely to be in white-collar jobs, so may be economically disadvantaged.

Turning to second generation Irish, there is evidence for upward mobility in occupation and education on their part in comparison to the English (Hornsby-Smith and Dale, cited in Harding and Balarajan, 1996). More second generation Irish (30% men, 39% women) are reported in non-manual social classes than all study members (25% men, 26% women) in a 1% sample of the population of England and Wales, mainly because of the larger proportion in class III non-manual (Harding and Balarajan, 1996).

Trends in marketing and retailing and the likely impact upon patterns of food choice.

We have referred to the changes in retailing in the Republic which resemble those in Britain. While Irish attitudes to food purchasing might be transferable on migration, the pattern of marketing and retailing in the Republic has no other implications for the Irish in Britain.

4. Research and intervention priorities

Practical suggestions on potential interventions, and enhancing the design of future dietary invention strategies

The lack of data concerning the nutritional status of Irish migrants to Britain and their descendants has directed the focus of this review on to studies from the Republic and Northern Ireland, since these could illuminate migrants' backgrounds, particularly the impact of their social class on their dietary practices. In the absence of basic data it is not possible to make suggestions about nutritional interventions particularly adapted to Irish migrants and their descendants, nor about ways of enhancing the design of interventions for this purpose, but it follows that the scope for research is considerable.

In the meantime, some nutritional interventions which are already standard may also be focused in the direction of the British-born with Irish ancestry:

- One area of concern is the short stature of descendants of Irish migrants in Britain, which is not apparent in surveys in Ireland, and is not explained by social class, though it may be explicable by additional indices of deprivation. Health professionals concerned with childhood growth in centres of current or former Irish migration should seek ways of monitoring children with Irish ancestry to identify phases of slow growth, and to ensure maximum uptake of rights to financial and nutritional support.

- There is a continuity between high rates for CHD and large bowel cancer in Ireland and in Irish migrants to Britain, which suggests that dietary interventions appropriate to reducing CHD in the British population generally may also appropriately be directed to those with Irish ancestry

Research priorities, including appropriate research questions

Basic research on the causes of excess mortality and morbidity in the descendants of Irish migrants to Britain is in progress but is not yet far advanced (Harding and Balarajan, 1996; Abbotts *et al.*, 1997). While basic research is not the Department of Health's primary role, it is appropriate under its nutrition priorities to encourage the collection or analysis of basic data sets:

- To relate Irish mortality and morbidity in Britain to data on childhood growth and nutritional circumstances.

- To relate Irish CHD risk in Britain to adult food choice and nutrient intakes.

Descriptive data are also needed on potential areas of concern for intervention:

- Basic data on growth and nutrient intakes of children with Irish ancestry in Britain would indicate the extent of any difficulties.

- Studies of dietary intake related to heart disease in areas of current or former Irish migration could clarify the extent of variation from recommended levels of intake by including indicators of Irish migration and ancestry.

- Research should focus not only on migrants, but also on their descendants in Britain, since several studies now show a continuing pattern (Raftery, Jones and Rosato, 1990; Harding and Balarajan. 1996; Abbotts *et al.*, 1997).

- Studies of the attitudes and beliefs of migrants about CHD may be indicated by evidence from the Republic of a lack of awareness of the incidence and prevalence of the disease, and of the potential for its prevention.

- Attention should be paid to the intake of dietary fat and fibre, given the high level of these intakes and the low level of exercise in Irish migrants to Boston, the apparent role of these nutrients in the aetiology of CHD, cancers of the digestive system and obesity, and the Irish evidence that men, and also women in economically inactive households, are more favourable to foods rich in these components.

● Further anthropometric data are required to clarify the prevalence of overweight and obesity, particularly centralised, in the Irish-descended population in Britain

Appendices

Appendix A. Study summary table

Abraham *et al.* (1985)
Harrow

Purpose
Descriptive

Design
Study type:
Data type: Quantitative
Data collection method: 7-day recall food intake
Sample type: Patient series (S. Asians) random ('European' controls)
Sample size: 813 South Asians
54 Europeans
Response rate:
Date study carried out: August 1977–November 1980

Comments
Hindu and Muslim women (women of other South Asian religions excluded)

Abraham *et al.* (1987)
Harrow

Purpose
Descriptive

Design
Study type:
Data type: Quantitative
Data collection method: 7-day recall food intake
Sample type: Patient series (S. Asians) random ('European' controls)
Sample size: 813 South Asians
54 Europeans
Response rate:
Date study carried out: August 1977–November 1980

Comments
Hindu and Muslim women (women of other South Asian religions excluded

Agha *et al.* (1992)
Islamabad

Purpose
Descriptive

Design
Study type:
Data type: Quantitative
Data collection method: Blood tests; no details of method used to gather background information
Sample type: Quota
Sample size: 270 (13–20 years)
Response rate:
Date study carried out:

Comments
Four Federal Government schools located in suburbs of Islamabad
170 boys (mean age 15.2)
100 girls (mean age 14.6)

Anderson and Lean (1995)
Glasgow

Purpose
Descriptive

Design
Study type:
Data type:
Data collection method: 7-day weighed intake diary
Sample type: Selective sub-sample from random sample
Sample size: 10
Response rate: 13 of 25
Date study carried out: 1993

Comments
8 Sikh, 2 Muslim women, mean age 54.2
Comparison of dietary habits of women in 1983 and 1993 but not designed as longitudinal study

Anon. (1986)
Republic of Ireland

Purpose
Descriptive

Design
Study type:
Data type: Qualitative
Data collection method: Interview
focus groups

Sample type: Opportunistic
Sample size: 39 women
Response rate:
Date study carried out:

Comments
Qualitative interviews: no further details.
17 Dublin women (20–54 years)
12 urban (non-Dublin) women (20–54)
12 rural women (20–54)
14 focus groups, age groups varied between 20–24 and
45–54

Armstrong (1989)
Sligo, North West Ireland

Purpose
Descriptive

Design
Study type:
Data type: Quantitative
Data collection method: Haematological tests only
Sample type: Quota
Sample size: 148 girls, 86 boys aged 14.5–18.4 (mean 15.9)
Response rate: 234/439
Date study carried out:

Comments
Short report
Five second-level schools

Barker et al. (1989)
Northern Ireland

Purpose
Descriptive

Design
Study type: Cross-sectional study
Data type: Quantitative
Data collection method: 7-day weighed intake diary; open,
structured questionnaire; anthropometrics
Sample type: Random, stratified
Sample size: 268 men, 348 women
Response rate: 77.3% (74.3% diaries)
Date study carried out: 1986–1987

Comments
Sample stratified by population density of 3 sub-regions in
Northern Ireland. Random selection of individuals from each
household using Kish sampling method.
Respondents aged 16–64

Barker et al. (1990)
Northern Ireland

Purpose
Explanatory (observational)

Design
Study type: Cross-sectional study
Data type: Quantitative
Data collection method: 7-day weighed intake diary; open,
structured questionnaire; anthropometrics
Sample type: Random, stratified
Sample size: 258 men, 334 women
Response rate: 77.3% (74.3% diaries)
Date study carried out: 1986–1987

Comments
Derived from study of diet, lifestyle and health in Northern
Ireland (Barker et al., 1989) but number of respondents does
not correspond.
Respondents aged 16–64

Barker, Thompson and McClean (1995)
Northern Ireland

Purpose
Explanatory (observational)

Design
Study type: Cross-sectional study
Data type: Quantitative
Data collection method: 7-day weighed intake diary; open,
structured questionnaire; anthropometrics
Sample type: Random, stratified
Sample size: 258 men, 334 women
Response rate: 77.3% (74.3% diaries)
Date study carried out: 1986–1987

Comments
Derived from study of diet, lifestyle and health in Northern
Ireland (Barker et al., 1989) but number of respondents does
not correspond.
Respondents aged 16–64

Bashir, Macdonald and Peacock (1981)
Leeds

Purpose
Descriptive

Design
Study type: Cross-sectional
Data type: Quantitative
Data collection method: Biochemical samples
Sample type: Patient series (ante-natal)
Sample size: 58 South Asian women
59 'Caucasian' controls
Response rate:
Date study carried out:

Comments

South Asian and 'Caucasian' controls matched for age, parity and gestational age.

South Asians not differentiated further

Beshyah, Jowett and Burden (1992)

Leicester

Purpose

Explanatory (observational)

Design

Study type: Longitudinal
Data type: Quantitative
Data collection method: Biochemical samples, weight
Sample type: Patient series (diabetic clinic)
Sample size: 7 men, 8 women
Response rate: 15/26*
Date study carried out:

Comments

Not stated if patient series selective or complete. Authors say sample not randomised because considered unethical on religious grounds to randomise to fasting/non-fasting groups.

Mean age 49.8 (range 21–71)

*Responding and intending to fast

Bhalla and Blakemore (1981)

Birmingham

Purpose

Descriptive

Design

Study type:
Data type: Quantitative
Data collection method: Open, structured interview; postal questionnaire survey (day centres)
Sample type: 'Door-to-door random sampling'
Sample size: 169 South Asian
179 African-Caribbean
52 'European'
Response rate:
Date study carried out: Began June 1979

Comments

Research carried out by MAFS (Market Research) Ltd with questionnaires provided by authors. Postal questionnaire surveyed day and social centres and old people's homes

84% South Asians were Indian

71% African-Caribbean were Jamaican

S. Asians: 107 men, 62 women

A. Caribbean: 68 men, 111 women

European: 17 men, 35 women

Age: 60 and over

Bhopal (1986a)

Glasgow

Purpose

Descriptive

Design

Study type:
Data type: Quantitative/qualitative
Data collection method: Interview*
Sample type: Random, stratified
Sample size: 65 South Asian
30 men, 35 women
Response rate: 67%
Date study carried out:

Comments

30 Muslim, 19 Sikh, 13 Hindu, 2 Christian and 1 atheist.

Median age 31 (range 19–70 years)

Family origin of all persons was NW of Indian sub-continent with majority from the Punjab; 55 respondents were migrant – median duration of residence 17 years (range 1–32)

*55 open questions

Boreham et al. (1993)

Northern Ireland

Purpose

Descriptive

Design

Study type:
Data type: Quantitative
Data collection method: Open, structured interview; diet history using photographic atlas to determine portion sizes
Sample type: Random, stratified
Sample size: 1015
Response rate: 78%
Date study carried out:

Comments

2% random sample of boys and girls of 12 and 15 years in Northern Ireland

Bose (1995)

Peterborough

Purpose

Descriptive

Design

Study type:
Data type: Quantitative
Data collection method: Not stated; anthropometrics
Sample type: Pakistani: patient series (complete)
'white': random from GP lists
Sample size: 100 Pakistani
262 'white'
Response rate: 'Approximately 25%'
Date study carried out:

Comments

Sample aged 20 or older

Box (1983)

Southall (West London)

Purpose
Explanatory (experimental)

Design
Study type: Before-and-after
Data type: Quantitative
Data collection method: Interview; diet history
Sample type: Patient series (ante-natal)*
Sample size: 20 South Asian
Response rate:
Date study carried out: January–April 1981

Comments
South Asians not differentiated but reference to 'Hindu, Muslim and Sikh language' abilities of clinic receptionists who 'could usually interpret' when necessary (1983, p. 132).
*Not clear if complete

Brooke and Wood (1980)

London

Purpose
Explanatory (observational)

Design
Study type: Longitudinal
Data type: Quantitative
Data collection method: Not specified; suite of physical measures
Sample type: Patient series*
Sample size: 80 South Asian infants
243 'white' infants
Response rate:
Date study carried out:

Comments
Weight, crown–heel length and head circumference measured at birth and at 3, 6, 9 and 12 months of age; origin of families of S. Asian infants: 73% from India (maj. Gujaratis and Punjabis), 17 % Pakistan, 10% Bangladesh, Sri Lanka or East Africa (Indian or Pakistan origin)
*'Unselected' (p. 355)

Brunvand et al. (1995)

Oslo

Purpose
Explanatory (observational)

Design
Study type: Cross-sectional
Data type: Quantitative
Data collection method: Diet history (Pakistani) self-administered food frequency questionnaire (Norwegian); biochemical assays and biochemical analysis of chapatti and bread material

Sample type: Patient series (ante-natal): Pakistani: complete Norwegian: selective
Sample size: 38 Pakistani, 38 Norwegian
Response rate: 68% Pakistani, 84% Norwegian
Date study carried out: 6 October 1991–15 January 1992

Comments
Pakistani women had been in Norway on average for five years (range 6 months to 15 years)

Burton-Jeangros (1995)

Cardiff

Purpose
Explanatory (observational)

Design
Study type: Cross-sectional
Data type: Quantitative
Data collection method: 'Semi-standardised questionnaire' (1995:66)
Sample type: Opportunistic
Sample size: 8 Pakistani women
Response rate:
Date study carried out: May–June 1993

Comments
No controls
17 women born in Pakistan, 1 British-born
2 women aged less than 20
10 women aged 20–29
6 women aged over 30

Campbell-Brown et al. (1985)

Harrow

Purpose
Explanatory (observational)

Design
Study type: *
Data type: Quantitative
Data collection method: 7-day dietary recall; description of foods eaten†
Sample type: Patient series (ante-natal): complete (Hindu) random (one in five) European
Sample size: 92 Hindu, 52 'Europeans'
Response rate: 69% Hindu
74% Europeans
Date study carried out: November 1979–June 1980

Comments
*Longitudinal measurements during pregnancy of zinc/copper concentrations in plasma/hair; dietary assessment cross-sectional
†Intake of 88 Hindus (96%), first 14 Europeans (27%) assessed by 7-day recall, remainder described foods they ate

Chandalia and Bhargav (1987)

Diabetes Clinic, J. J. Hospital and Grant Medical College
Bombay

Purpose

Explanatory (experimental)

Design

Study type: Before-and-after
Data type: Quantitative
Data collection method: Detailed diet history using 'oral
questionnaire method' p. 287*
Sample type: Patient series
Sample size: 13 Muslims
Response rate:
Date study carried out:

Comments

Elicited information on economic/living conditions, food
habits and common dietary pattern, methods of cooking,
food sharing practices, total daily consumption of various
food items in family; daily per capita consumptions of various
foods and their nutritive value.
*Recorded 2–5 days prior to Ramadan

Clarson et al. (1982)

Sorrento Maternity Hospital, Birmingham

Purpose

Explanatory (observational)

Design

Study type: Cross-sectional*
Data type: Quantitative
Data collection method: Derived from clinical records
Sample type: Patient series (selective)
Sample size: Indian (1968) 106
Indian (1978) 70
Pakistani (1968) 152
Pakistani (1978) 228
Response rate: Not applicable
Date study carried out: Not applicable

Comments

1968: 106 Indian, 152 Pakistani mothers
1978: 70 Indians, 202 Pakistanis, 26 Bangladeshi
(Pakistani/Bangladeshi combined for comparisons with
Indians, and examination of secular change)
*At two time points (1968, 1978)

Cross, Eminson and Wharton (1990)

Birmingham

Purpose

Explanatory (observational)

Design

Study type:
Data type: Quantitative
Data collection method: Derived from birth data for

Birmingham 1964–1984
Sample type: Patient series (complete)
Sample size: 13 351 S. Asian Muslim
13 351 white
5106 S. Asian non-Muslim
Response rate: Not applicable
Date study carried out: Not applicable

Comments

Each S. Asian Muslim baby was matched with a white and a
S. Asian non-Muslim baby born within two days of the Muslim
birth to control for secular and seasonal changes in
distribution of birthweights. It was not always possible to
select a non-Muslim control because a birth in this group did
not always occur within two days of a Muslim birth.

Davies et al. (1982)

Leicester

Purpose

Descriptive

Design

Study type:
Data type: Quantitative
Data collection method: Physical measures (infants)*
Sample type: I: random sample from birth series
II: 20 full-term South Asian babies; 20 full-term white babies†
Sample size: I:50 South Asian mothers and babies; 50 white
mothers and babies
II: see sample type
Response rate:
Date study carried out: I: February–March 1979
II: February–May 1979

Comments

Comparison of results from two studies designed
independently, hence designs differ
South Asians not differentiated further. South Asian mothers:
mean age 25
White mothers: mean age 26
*Waist–hip ratio as indicator of maternal nutritional status
†Babies not matched; sampling method not clear

Dhawan (1995)

Bolton District General Hospital

Purpose

Descriptive

Design

Study type: Retrospective case note study
Data type: Quantitative
Data collection method: Derived from obstetric notes
Sample type: Random selection from patient series*
Sample size: 331 South Asian
Response rate: Not applicable
Date study carried out: Not applicable

Comments

220 women born on Indian sub-continent

111 British-born South Asian

S. Asians were not reported as differentiated to sub-group

*Women who gave birth between January and December 1989

Duggan et al. (1991)

Sheffield

Purpose

Descriptive

Design

Study type:

Data type: Quantitative

Data collection method: 4-day weighed dietary inventory*; anthropometrics; haematological investigations

Sample type: Sample of child health and GP clinic populations

Sample size: 138 South Asian infants

Response rate:

Date study carried out: 12-month period, year unstated

Comments

97 of 138 completed dietary inventory. Selection methods not clear: 'recruited over a 12-month period from the registers of the nine child health and general practitioner clinics which serve the majority of the Asian community' p. 1386. Sample aged 4–40 months, not reported as differentiated to sub-groups but S. Asians in Sheffield are largely Muslim

*5 days for children older than 12 months

Duggan et al. (1992)

Sheffield

Purpose

Explanatory (observational)

Design

Study type: Cross-sectional

Data type: Quantitative

Data collection method: Weighed dietary inventory*

Sample type: Sample of child health and GP clinic populations and also opportunistic†

Sample size: 195 families

Response rate: 58%

Date study carried out: February 1989–February 1990

Comments

Sample aged 4–40 months, not reported as differentiated to sub-groups, but S. Asians in Sheffield are largely Muslim. 154 weighed dietary studies completed in twelve-month period

*3 days in children < 12 months; 5 days in older children.

†437 Asian babies registered at clinics were targeted for recruitment; 21 children aged 24 months or more were recruited in the field

Eaton, Wharton and Wharton (1984)

Sorrento Maternity Hospital, Birmingham

Purpose

Descriptive

Design

Study type:

Data type: Quantitative

Data collection method: 3-day weighed intake, plus 24-hour recall*

Sample type: Patient series†

Sample size: 89 South Asian women

Response rate:

Date study carried out: January–November, year unstated

Comments

Style of reporting makes ascertainment of sample size and methodology problematic.

*3 weekday weighed intakes at 18, 23, 28, 33, 38 weeks of every 5th women taking part in supplement trial (see Viegas et al., 1982a and b). Intakes of other women recalled once in each trimester at 23 and 33 weeks: weighed intakes: 17, recalled intakes 72

†Booked before 20 weeks gestation and living within defined area of city of Birmingham

Ebrahim et al. (1991)

North London

Purpose

Explanatory (observational)

Design

Study type: Cross-sectional

Data type: Quantitative

Data collection method: Administered interview schedule;* anthropometrics and other medical assessment

Sample type: S. Asian: patient series (complete) non-S. Asian: patient series (selective)†

Sample size: S. Asian: 59
non-S. Asian: 59

Response rate: S. Asian: 82%, non-S. Asian: 88%

Date study carried out:

Comments

Respondents aged 55+

Mean age: S. Asians 62.9, non-S. Asian 63.9

42% of respondents were female (25 per group)

*No further details

†Matched against each S. Asian subject selected at random from age–sex register of general practice

Ehrhardt (1985)

Bradford

Purpose

Descriptive

Design

Study type:

Data type: Quantitative

Data collection method: Haematological tests

Sample type: Patient series (complete)*

Sample size: 265 S. Asian children
513 'white' children

Response rate:

Date study carried out: Not applicable

Comments

No dietary data recorded

*Paediatric admissions 1.9.83–29.2.84; eligible if at least 6 months of age and less than 4 years on date of admission; children admitted more than once were studied during the initial admission. 14 of 792 children excluded on medical grounds or because of other ethnic minorities

Evans *et al.* (1995)

Belfast and Toulouse

Purpose

Comparative descriptive

Design

Study type:
Data type: Quantitative
Data collection method: Belfast: 3 day-weighed intake Toulouse: 3-day food diaries (400), and 3-day precise weighed intake
Sample type: Stratified random
Sample size: Belfast: 401 men
Toulouse: 400 men
Response rate: Diaries:
Belfast 52%
Toulouse 58%
Date study carried out: Belfast 1985–86
Toulouse

Comments

For each Toulouse subject, two Belfast subjects were selected by matching for height, weight and age.
Dietary analysis restricted to 40 weighed intakes (Toulouse) and 80 weighed intakes (Belfast)

Finch, Millard and Maxwell (1991)

Chest clinic of St James' Hospital, Balham, South London

Purpose

Explanatory (observational)

Design

Study type: Cross-sectional
Data type: Quantitative
Data collection method: Case notes
Sample type: Total patient series *
Sample size: 620 S. Asian†
432 'UK whites'
Response rate: Not applicable
Date study carried out: Not applicable

Comments

*Records of all patients diagnosed with TB between 1973–1988 were reviewed; all S. Asian migrants from India, Pakistan and East Africa with TB compared with 'white' patients born in UK
†420 Hindu, 151 Muslim, 49 other religions

Finch *et al.* (1992)

St George's Hospital, Wandsworth, South London

Purpose

Explanatory (observational)

Design

Study type: Cross-sectional
Data type: Quantitative
Data collection method: Food frequency dietary score; blood samples; bone biopsy
Sample type: Patient series*
Sample size:
175 S. Asians
Response rate:
Date study carried out:

Comments

*New attenders at general medical OP clinic (not referred with possible metabolic bone disease or vitamin D deficiency); recruited over a 2-year period
77 males; 98 non-pregnant females; 67 (26%) Hindu.
56 bone biopsies of 62 considered at risk of osteomalacia

Ford *et al.* (1972)

Glasgow

Purpose

Descriptive

Design

Study type:
Data type: Quantitative
Data collection method: Administered interview schedule*; blood samples
Sample type: 1. opportunistic 2. patient series†
Sample size: 1. 26 S. Asian households (115 people)
Response rate: 52% (26 of 50 households)
Date studied carried out: April–May 1971

Comments

*Interview carried out in respondents' homes, no details of schedule structure
†Data on admissions to all Glasgow hospitals of children with diagnosis of rickets (1968–70)

Fowler *et al.* (1990)

Dudley Road Hospital, Birmingham

Purpose

Explanatory (observational)

Design

Study type: Retrospective
Data type: Quantitative
Data collection method: Analysis of clinic attendance records; self-complete questionnaires*
Sample type: 2 patient series
Sample size: 78 Muslim women
Response rate:†
Date study carried out: 6 March–6 April 1989
(pre-Ramadan)
7 April–8 May 1989 (Ramadan)

Comments

Comparison of antenatal clinic attendance during Ramadan (1989) with similar time-span outside Ramadan, for Muslim and non-Muslim women

*Questionnaires completed prior to Ramadan regarding observation of Ramadan fast by Muslim women attending ante-natal clinic and intention to attend clinic during Ramadan

†Text implies 100% since 78 women who completed questionnaires described as 'consecutive' but no other details of sampling given

Gibney and Lee (1989)

Kilkenny, Southern Ireland

Purpose
Descriptive

Design
Study type:
Data type: Quantitative
Data collection method: 7-day weighed intake
Sample type: Stratified random*
Sample size: 30 male, 30 female
Response rate:
Date study carried out: June–August 1985

Comments
*Subjects randomly selected from 332 individuals (aged 35–44) who were initially randomly selected from the electoral register

Gishen, Hogh and Stock (1995)

St George's Hospital Medical School, London

Purpose
Descriptive

Design
Study type:
Data type: Quantitative
Data collection method: Anthropometrics
Sample type: *
Sample size: S. Asian 60 male, 34 female, European male 115, female 121
Response rate:
Date study carried out:

Comments
*†The sampling method is unclear. Subjects are medical students whose anthropometrics were recorded for two earlier research projects in 1991 and 1994. 28% of students at this medical school are S. Asian, but not clear if all took part. Mean age: SA male 19.7, female 19.2, European male 19.6, female 19.5: not significantly different

Griffiths (1983)

Birmingham

Purpose
Descriptive

Design
Study type:
Data type: Quantitative
Data collection method: Self-complete schedule
Sample type: Opportunistic
Sample size: West Indian families: 142
Indian families: 146
Pakistani families: 139
Response rate: West Indian: 71%
Indian: 73%
Pakistani 70%
Date study carried out:

Comments
No details of structure of interview schedule
No description of sampling strategy

Grindulis *et al.* (1986)

Birmingham

Purpose
Explanatory (observational)

Design
Study type: Cross-sectional
Data type: Quantitative
Data collection method: Diet history, clinical examination, anthropometry, blood tests, psychomotor development assessment
Sample type: Patient series
Sample size: S. Asian: 145
Response rate:
Date study carried out:

Comments
Infants (21–23 months) who had been born at Sorrento Maternity Hospital; mothers had taken part in study of nutritional supplementation in pregnancy (Viegas *et al.*, 1982 a and b)
No controls

Harbottle and Duggan (1992)

Sheffield

Purpose
Explanatory (observational)

Design
Study type: Cross-sectional
Data type: Quantitative
Data collection method: Weighed dietary inventory
Sample type: Sample of child health and GP clinic populations and also opportunistic
Sample size: 32 S. Asian infants
Response rate: Not applicable
Date study carried out: Not applicable

Comments
Analysis of sub-set of data described in Duggan *et al.* (1992); original data collected over a 12-month period
12 iron-deficient infants

20 'normal' infants
Aged 4–40 months; not differentiated to sub-groups

Harding and Balarajan (1996)

Purpose
Explanatory (observational)

Design
Study type: Longitudinal
Data type: Quantitative
Data collection method: Drawn from 1971 census
Sample type: 1% random sample of population of England and Wales
Sample size: 3075 men; 3233 women
Response rate:
Date study carried out:

Comments
Sample aged 15 and over in 1971
Deaths analysed in follow-up period 1971–1989

Harris et al. (1983)

Purpose
Descriptive

Design
Study type:
Data type: Quantitative
Data collection method: 7-day diet history;* administered questionnaire
Sample type: Random
Sample size: 76 Bangladeshi babies
Response rate:
Date study carried out: 6-month period – no dates

Comments
No details of questionnaire structure
Sample chosen at random by health visitors over 6-month period; no controls
60 aged 6–12 months, 76 aged 1–2 years, 23 aged 2–3 years, 18 aged 3–5 years
*Estimation of quantities based on household measures

Henderson et al. (1989)

Glasgow

Purpose
Explanatory (experimental)

Design
Study type: Before-and-after
Data type: Quantitative
Data collection method: Administered questionnaires; pre- and post-campaign surveys of prevalence of osteomalacia by blood test
Sample type: Opportunistic;* random†
Sample size: 1st questionnaire: 252
2nd questionnaire 188

blood test 1) 203 women
blood test 2) 59 women
Response rate:
Date study carried out: 1st questionnaire September 1984
2nd questionnaire March 1985; blood tests January–March 982–1983, 1986

Comments
Testing attitudes of Asian women to vitamin D self-supplementation
First questionnaire respondents were visited May–August 1984 by linkworkers to explain campaign and to sell supplements; emphasis on Sikh and Hindu families.
Second questionnaire completed with women who had completed first. Assessed attitudes to supplement purchase and self-administration six months after home sales of supplements had been withdrawn
Second paired blood sample provided in 1986 by 59 women aged 23–60 (median 37 years) from one of general practices in 1982–83 study, and by 80 women aged 17–47 (median 26 years) attending 3 health board clinics with their children
*List of Asian households obtained from voters' rolls in city's libraries
†Blood samples provided by 203 women aged 19–60 (median 33 years) randomly sampled from age–sex registers of 3 general practices

Henderson et al. (1990)

Glasgow

Purpose
Explanatory (observational)

Design
Study type: Case-control
Data type: Quantitative
Data collection method: 7-day weighed dietary intake (91) recall (13); 7-day record of daylight outdoor exposure; bloods
Sample type: Patient series (cases) sample of general practice population (controls)
Sample size: 27 cases,* 77 controls
Response rate: 60%
Date study carried out: 1982–1985

Comments
Cases = S. Asian women discharged from all Glasgow hospitals (1972–1984) with diagnosis of privational osteomalacia; controls = S. Asian women part of random sample drawn from 3 inner-city GP practices (Henderson et al., 1989); respondents mainly Pakistani Muslim
Weighed intakes 91 (19 cases, 72 controls), recalls 12 (8 cases 5 controls)
*Includes 5 with biochemical evidence of osteomalacia originally recruited as controls

Henriksen et al. (1995)

Aker and Ullevål University Hospitals, Oslo, Norway

Purpose
Explanatory (observational)

Design
Study type: Cross-sectional

Data type: Quantitative
Data collection method: Questionnaire; 24-hr recall;
administered food questionnaire*
Sample type: Pakistani: patient series (complete)†
Norwegian: random selection from patient series
Sample size: Pakistani: 38
Norwegian: 38
Response rate: Pakistani: 66%
Norwegian: 84%
Date study carried out: October 1991–January 1992

Comments
No details of questionnaire structure
*Containing 120 Pakistani foods/dishes and covering usual intake with
previous month as reference. Portion sizes estimated. Snacks and
common foods eaten between meals recorded. Norwegians: self-
complete food frequency questionnaire, and portion size estimation
†Women referred for ultrasound were surveyed at 18 weeks of
pregnancy

Hilder (1994)

East London districts (Hackney, Tower Hamlets, Newham)

Purpose
Explanatory (observational)

Design
Study type: Retrospective
Data type: Quantitative
Data collection method: Analysis of obstetric/child health
data
Sample type: Patient series*
Sample size: 39 101 births†
Response rate: Not applicable
Date study carried out: Not applicable

Comments
Mothers: 17 780 Anglo-European; 6219 Bangladeshi origin;
3598 Indian; 1602 Pakistani; 3016 West Indian; 3073 African,
3813 other ethnic groups. Matched with 312 death
registration records to validate death and add registered
cause of death
Mortality rates calculated in usual way, and using life-table
methods
*Assumed complete – not stated explicitly
†Born 1989–1990

Homans (1983)

Coventry

Purpose
Descriptive

Design
Study type:
Data type: Qualitative
Data collection method: Interviews (2)*
Sample type: Patient series, ante-natal clinic (no other
details)
Sample size: 39 S. Asian migrants
39 British

Response rate:
Date study carried out: 1976–1979

Comments
*Two interviews: 1. at first visit to ante-natal clinic 2. 26 women
from both groups given 'long structured interview' at home
when 8 months pregnant, using interpreter as necessary. No
other details of structure; both interviews included dietary
questions
S. Asians not differentiated

Iqbal *et al.* (1994)

Leicester General Hospital, Leicester

Purpose
Descriptive

Design
Study type:
Data type: Quantitative
Data collection method: Biochemical tests and bone biopsy
Sample type: Patient series
Sample size: 26 S. Asians
Response rate:
Date study carried out:*

Comments
Not clear if this is a complete patient series and if all patients
were migrant; ages ranged from 2 months to 61 years (3
younger than 15: 1 aged 6–15, 2 less than 1 year)
23 patients 'were Hindu or from Hindu families who were
vegetarians' (p. 711)
*Report describes patients who presented medically over a
consecutive period of three and a half years (no dates)

Irish Nutrition and Dietetic Institute (1990)

Republic of Ireland

Purpose
Descriptive

Design
Study type:
Date type: Quantitative
Data collection method: 7-day diet history; questionnaire;*
anthropometrics
Sample type: Random
Sample size: 1214
Response rate:
Date study carried out: 1989

Comments
*For respondents' background – no details of structure given
Photographic atlas used to estimate portion sizes
538 aged 8–18 years, 676 aged 18 years or older

Jones (1987)

Tower Hamlets, East London

Purpose

Descriptive

Design

Study type:
Date type: Quantitative
Data collection method: Administered questionnaire
Sample type: Patient series, ante-natal*
Sample size: 25 Bangladeshi, 25 'East Berkshire'
Response rate:
Date study carried out: 1985

Comments

No details of questionnaire structure; description of methodology lacks detail
*Women attending ante-natal clinics in second or subsequent pregnancy randomly selected
Bangladeshi mean age 27 (range 18–38)
East Berkshire mean age 29 (range 21–40)

Kalka (1988)

Harrow, North London

Purpose

Descriptive

Design

Study type:
Date type: Qualitative
Data collection method:
Sample type:
Sample size:*
Response rate:
Date study carried out: 1984, 1986 (Gujarat)

Comments

Study of food habits in Gujarati families in Harrow, and occasional comparison to habits in Gujarat studied in two field visits. No information regarding data collection method, sample type, response rate
*Refers to data on breakfast menus obtained from 57 women interviewed in Northwick Park Hospital ante-natal clinic – no other indication of possible sample source or size

Kassam-Khamis *et al.* (1995)

Southall, Brent and Wembley, London

Purpose

Descriptive

Design

Study type:
Data type: Quantitative
Data collective method: 1. & 2.: 7-day weighed intake
3. 5-day weighed intake
Sample type:
Sample size: 1. 92 S. Asian men*

2. 23 Gujarati women
3. 20 Gujarati men
Response rate:
Date study carried out: 1. 1989; 2. 1987; 3, year unknown

Comments

Frequency of consumption of 'traditional' dishes and recipe details taken from 2 published studies and 1 unpublished study
*1. 88/92 were Punjabi Sikhs (Southall)
2. Vegetarian, pre-menopausal Gujaratis (Brent)
3. Gujaratis (Wembley), as part of the Wembley Coronary Heart Disease Study

Kearney and Gibney (1993)

1. Republic of Ireland

Purpose

Explanatory (observational)

Design

Study type: Cross-sectional
Data type: Quantitative
Data collection method: 'Structured, interview-assisted questionnaire'
Sample type: Stratified random*
Sample size: 1400
Response rate:
Date study carried out:

Comments

Abstract only, therefore few details
*Baseline survey of 'a nationally representative, quota-controlled (for gender, age, social class and region) sample' 'aged 15 years plus'

Kearney and Gibney (1993)

2. Greater Dublin area

Purpose

Explanatory (observational)

Design

Study type: Case-control
Data type: Quantitative
Data collection method: 7-day diet history;* interview-assisted questionnaire†
Sample type: Quota‡
Sample size: 40 users (34 female, 6 male), 40 non-users
Response rate:
Date study carried out:

Comments

Abstract only, therefore few details
*Aided by photographic food atlas
†27 questions on nutritional knowledge
‡'From a sample of 175 supplement users, recruited in health food shops in the Greater Dublin area, 40 were selected who could be classified as '"heavy" users'. Matched with controls for age, gender and educational status

Kemm, Douglas and Sylvester (1986)

Birmingham

Purpose
Descriptive

Design
Study type:
Data type: Quantitative
Data collection method: Structured interview;* household food consumption patterns (102); food diaries (78)
Sample type:
Sample size: 131 African-Caribbean mothers of male infants, aged 18–41
Response rate:
Date study carried out:

Comments
†57% born in UK; main age of entry to UK of remainder was 13 years
89/131 in 'stable union'
75/131 on supplementary benefit
*Obtained socioeconomic and demographic data; breast-feeding and weaning data; sources of information about infant feeding

Kelleher and Islam (1994)

Tower Hamlets, East London

Purpose
Descriptive

Design
Study type:
Data type: Qualitative
Data collection method: Taped interviews, supplemented by observation*
Sample type: Quota
Sample size: 40 Bangladeshi migrants†
25 men, 15 women
Response rate:
Date study carried out:

Comments
All interviews except 2 conducted in Sylheti dialect and translated into English
30 close relatives also interviewed
†Article reports preliminary analysis of 12 diabetic men and 8 diabetic women; 8 under 50 years of age, 12 over 50 years
*Of research assistant who lives in this community

Khajuria and Thomas (1992)

London (diabetic clinics of two unnamed hospitals)

Purpose
Descriptive

Design
Study type:
Data type: Quantitative

Data collection method: Questionnaire; 24-hr recall food/drink
Sample type: Random sample from patient series
Sample size: 28 (8 men, 20 women)
Response rate:
Date study carried out:

Comments
Structure of interview questions not described
Interview (30–40 minutes) conducted in 'mixture of Gujarati and English' (p. 314)
16 < 54 years of age, 12 aged 55–75

Knight et al. (1992)

Bradford

Purpose
Explanatory (observational)

Design
Study type: Cross-sectional
Data type: Quantitative
Data collection method: Food frequency questionnaire, 3-day diet diary (not specified if weighed); anthropometrics, bloods
Sample type: Quota*
Sample size: S. Asian men: 110; non-S. Asian men: 156
Response rate: S. Asian: 84%; non-S. Asian: 71%
Date study carried out:

Comments
Aged 20–65
63.5% Muslim (Pakistani or Punjabi)
31.3% Hindu
5.2% Sikh/not stated (not presented in report because of small number)
*'Within one socioeconomic stratum' in two textile factories (p. 343)

Kushi et al. (1985)

Republic of Ireland and Boston, USA

Purpose
Explanatory (observational)

Design
Study type: Prospective cohort
Data type: Quantitative
Data collection method: Food frequency constructed from diet history
Sample type: Quota
Sample size: Boston brothers: 563 (390)
Irish brothers: 572 (386); Boston men born of Irish parents: 373 (225)
Response rate: 66%
Date study carried out: *

Comments
Figures in parentheses indicates number at follow-up
*Study began late 1959, Boston men of Irish parents enrolled 1959–65, 'vital status' of total of 3 cohorts (i.e. 1508) determined in 1982

Landman and Wyke (1995)
Edinburgh, Stirling, Glasgow

Purpose
Descriptive

Design
Study type:
Data type: Qualitative
Data collection method: Semi-structured interviews; focus groups
Sample type: Opportunistic
Sample size: 93 S. Asian men and women*
Response rate:
Date study carried out: Focus groups: July–Sept 1994
Interviews: October–November 1994

Comments
*48 at 6 focus groups, 45 interviews
25 Edinburgh, 19 Stirling, 49 Glasgow
30 British-born, 29 born in India, 22 born in Pakistan, 12 born elsewhere
48 'mothers', 15 'fathers', 30 young people
30 aged < 19, 14 aged 20–29, 34 aged 30–39, 15 aged > 40

Lip et al. (1995)
Birmingham

Purpose
Descriptive

Design
Study type:
Data type: Quantitative
Data collection method: Not explicit
Sample type: Random within patient series*
Sample size: 84 'white'
76 African-Caribbean
72 South Asian
Response rate:
Date study carried out: 4-month period (no date)

Comments
*Sample of pregnant women, no details of sampling procedure
White mean age 25.7
African-Caribbean mean age 24.7
S. Asian mean age 24.3

Lowry and Lillis (1993)
West of Ireland

Purpose
Descriptive

Design
Study type:
Data type: Quantitative
Data collection method: Interviews (no details)
Sample type: 1. patient series (ante-natal)

2. random*
Sample size: 1. 870 mothers
2. 103 breast-feeding
3. 170 bottle-feeding
Response rate:
Date study carried out: 1. August–December 1987
2. April 1988
3. June 1988

Comments
*Two separate follow-up surveys of breast-feeding and bottle feeding mothers

Mangtani et al. (1995)
32 London boroughs

Purpose
Explanatory (observational)

Design
Study type: Ecological analysis
Data type: Quantitative
Data collection method: Sociodemographic measures (1981 and 1991 censuses), tuberculosis notification rates (1982–91)
Sample type: Total patient series
Sample size:
Response rate: Not applicable
Date study carried out:

Mason, Davies and Marshall (1982)
Leicester Royal Infirmary Maternity Hospital

Purpose
Descriptive

Design
Study type:
Data type: Quantitative
Data collection method: Birthweight; weight at 2 months collected at clinic
Sample type: Total patient series
Sample size: 34 South Asian infants*
34 white infants
Response rate:
Date study carried out:

Comments
Infants born at term to Asian women (mainly Gujarati) who had not had complications in pregnancy which might have influenced intrauterine growth
Each baby was matched with a white term infant, born within 24 hours and same sex
*20 from East Africa, 14 from India

McFadyen et al. (1984)
Northwick Park Hospital, Harrow

Purpose
Explanatory (observational)

Design
Study type: Cross-sectional
Data type: Quantitative
Data collection method:*
Sample type: S. Asians: patient series; Europeans:†
Sample size: 664 Hindu babies
132 Muslim babies
486 European babies
Response rate:
Date study carried out: Births between 1977–1981

Comments
*Mother's country of birth, religion and husband's occupation recorded in addition to routine maternal/foetal observations, outcome of pregnancy, birthweight
†S. Asians unselected consecutive bookings; Europeans 'first two who attended the same ante-natal booking clinics over the same period of time' (p. 968). Hindus and Muslims from India, Pakistan, East Africa

McKeigue, Shah and Marmot (1991)
London

Purpose
Explanatory (observational)

Design
Study type: Cross-sectional
Data type: Quantitative
Data collection method: Self-complete; BP, anthropometrics, blood glucose
Sample type: Quota
Sample size: 1712 S. Asian
1761 non-S. Asian
Response rate: 62% S. Asian
66% non-S. Asian
Date study carried out: June 1988–July 1990

Comments
Sampled from 4 factories and 16 general practices (women from 3 of latter)
52% Sikh, 11% Punjabi Hindu, 9% Gujarati Hindu, 15% Muslim, 13% other
S. Asian: 291 women, 1421 men
Non-S. Asian: 246 women, 1515 men
209 African-Caribbean (partial analysis)
Men aged 40–64; women no age given

McNeil (1985)
Punjab, North India; West Midlands (no further details)

Purpose
Explanatory (observational)

Design
Study type: Cross-sectional
Data type: Quantitative
Data collection method: Interview (not described); physical measures
Sample type: See comments

Sample size: 78 UK Punjabi children
74 rural Punjabi children
Response rate:
Date study carried out:

Comments
Sampling method of rural Punjabi children not described – may be total sample – children were seen on regular home visits by staff of a rural health centre
Birthweights available for 39/74 rural Punjabi children and 71/78 UK Punjabi children who were all born in an unnamed West Midlands maternity hospital

McSweeney and Kevany (1982)
31 maternity units, Republic of Ireland

Purpose
Descriptive

Design
Study type:
Data type: Quantitative
Data collection method: Self-complete questionnaire*
Sample type: Patient series
Sample size: 31 units, 1195 mothers
Response rate: 100% (units)
Date study carried out: 27 April–4 May, year unstated

Comments
*Sent to matron/obstetrical consultant in each hospital for data relating to discharges from their unit during survey week; report sheet completed for each mother

Miller et al. (1988)
North West London

Purpose
Descriptive

Design
Study type:
Data type: Quantitative
Data collection method: Administered interview;* dietary intake
Sample type: Quota
Sample size: 75 Indian;† 64 European, 24 West Indian men
Response rate: 81% 'minimal estimate' (p. 65)
Date study carried out:

Comments
20 each European and Indian men who completed 1st part of study randomly sampled, plus 11 West Indian (not random); each completed a questionnaire of usual eating habits, and completed 5-day weighed dietary inventory
Sample aged 45–54; 81% of men registered with GP practice and registered within defined area
*No details of schedule structure given
†59 born India, 14 born East Africa, 2 born elsewhere; West Indians largely from Jamaica

Mulliner, Spiby and Fraser (1995)
Trent Region

Purpose
Descriptive

Design
Study type:
Data type: Qualitative and quantitative
Data collection method: 1. questionnaire*
2. semi-structured interview schedule
Sample type: Random†
Sample size: 58 midwives
Response rate: 78% including pilot study
Date study carried out:

Comments
†Sample of 77 midwives (10% of those in Trent Region)
selected using multi-stage random sampling technique; of the
ten maternity units approached, one was used for the pilot study
*For 'more factual information' (p. 38) e.g. education in nutrition since
registration; followed by interview for developing responses to
questionnaire

Nelson, Bakaliou and Trivedi (1994)
Wembley, Middlesex

Purpose
Explanatory (observational)

Design
Study type:
Data type: Quantitative
Data collection method: 1. postal questionnaires
2. self-complete*
Sample type: Quota
Sample size: 114 girls,† aged 11–14
Response rate: 37% (114 of 305 eligible)
Date study carried out:

Comments
Parents sent postal questionnaire re ethnic origin,
occupation, household composition, daughter's history of
infection
†37 white, 8 African-Caribbean, 58 Indian, 8 Pakistani,
3 other
*By respondents on eating habits, menstruation and habitual activity
levels; height/weight; 2 min. step test, blood test also taken

O'Reilly and Shelley (1991)
County Kilkenny, Republic of Ireland

Purpose
Descriptive

Design
Study type:
Data type: Quantitative
Data collection method: Self-complete questionnaire*
Sample type: Stratified random

Sample size: 228 boys, 217 girls
Response rate: 95%
Date study carried out: Spring 1987

Comments
*Developed from WHO core questionnaire
to determine knowledge, attitudes and behaviour relevant to
non-communicable diseases
Age range 11–19; 88% were aged 13–17; males and females
were equally represented

Ormerod *et al.* (1991)
Blackburn

Purpose
Comparative descriptive

Design
Study type:
Data type: Quantitative
Data collection method: Analysis of tuberculosis
notifications
Sample type: Patient series
Sample size: Blackburn 325 Indian, 309 Pakistani/
Bangladeshi
MRC Survey 674 Indian
348 Pakistani/Bangladeshi
Response rate: Not applicable
Date study carried out:

Comments
Study of disease characteristics of all TB patients in
Blackburn DHA for 1978–1987 compared with MRC survey –
all TB notifications in England and Wales for last six months of
1983

Potts and Simmons (1994)
Oxford Polytechnic, Oxford

Purpose
Explanatory (observational)

Design
Study type: Case-control
Data type: Quantitative
Data collection method:*
Sample type: Opportunistic†
Sample size: 80 S. Asian cases
80 'Europid' controls
Response rate: Not applicable
Date study carried out: October–December 1988

Comments
40 male, 40 female S. Asians and Europids, aged 20–23
93% UK-born, 7% lived in UK for a minimum of 14 years
Not differentiated to sub-groups
*'General questions were asked concerning subjects' diets' (p. 837)
†Students 'asked to volunteer' (p. 837)

Riddoch *et al.* (1991)
Northern Ireland

Purpose
Descriptive

Design
Study type:
Data type: Quantitative
Data collection method: Self-complete lifestyle questionnaire (supervisor assisted where necessary); anthropometry, fitness, physical activity
Sample type: Stratified random
Sample size: 1540 boys, 1671 girls
Response rate: (All) 72% boys, 75% girls
Date study carried out:

Comments
Random selection of 20 schools in Northern Ireland (from total of 256) chosen to provide widest range of pupils in each age/sex group
3211 children (1.25% of age population) were tested; age range 11–18; results for 17- to 18-year-olds not necessarily representative since most children of this age do not attend school

Robertson *et al.* (1982)
Glasgow

Purpose
Explanatory (observational)

Design
Study type: Cross-sectional
Data type: Quantitative
Data collection method: 7-day weighed dietary survey
Sample type:
Sample size: 84 S. Asian children
Response rate:
Date study carried out:

Comments
Subjects aged 8–16; not differentiated by sub-group
Minimal methodological details because it was planned to publish the study in more detail, but the reviewers were not able to trace a later publication

Rona *et al.* (1987)
National Study of Health and Growth

Purpose
Explanatory (observational)

Design
Study type: Cross-sectional
Data type: Quantitative
Data collection method: Self-complete questionnaire;* anthropometrics
Sample type: 1. stratified random

2. sample from inner city electoral wards†
Sample size: 381 'Urdu'‡ children p. 233
477 Gujarati children
1067 Punjabi children
Response rate:
Date study carried out: 1983

Comments
*On family social circumstances, child's wellbeing (including question asking if child is vegetarian and, if so, if dairy products are consumed
†With high proportions born in New Commonwealth (America and Asia) – sampling method not described
Sample age in 1983 not reported
‡Urdu is a language rather than a sub-national group, but Urdu-speakers are predominantly from Pakistan

Sahota (1991)
Bradford (3 inner city baby clinics)

Purpose
Descriptive

Design
Study type:
Data type: Quantitative
Data collection method: Questionnaire*
Sample type: Random
Sample size: 43 S. Asian women
29 European women
Response rate:
Date study carried out: March 1987

Comments
*Survey design unclear; questionnaire example is 'closed' but not clear if self-complete or administered – assumed latter since 15% of respondents reported to be illiterate. No details of sampling method
88% Pakistani, 7% Indian, 5% Bangladeshi (combined for analysis and discussion); infants of mothers were aged 3–18 months

Samanta *et al.* (1986)
Leicester (GP diabetic clinic)

Purpose
Descriptive

Design
Study type:
Data type: Quantitative
Data collection method: Food frequency questionnaire;* interview†
Sample type: Patient series
Sample size: 40
Response rate: 68% (40 of 59 attenders)
Date study carried out:

Comments
Study described in referenced letter to journal

Sample not differentiated by ethnic sub-group
*Average intake estimated from bulk buying, and number of heads per household.
†No details except 'in presence of a dietitian and doctor speaking appropriate language'; structure not described

Sevak, McKeigue and Marmot (1994)
Ealing, West London

Purpose
Explanatory (observational)

Design
Study type: Cross-sectional
Data type: Quantitative
Data collection method: 7-day weighed intakes
Sample type: Random, stratified by insulin levels
Sample size: S. Asian: 92
European: 81
Response rate: S. Asian: 59%*
European: 55%
Date study carried out:

Comments
Age 40–69 years
Successful dietary records completed by:
S.Asian low insulin group: 29
       intermediate group: 31
       high insulin group: 32
European low insulin group: 26
       intermediate group: 22
       high insulin group: 33
*At time of invitation to participate in diet survey, having been examined in main survey (McKeigue, Shah and Marmot, 1991)

Shahjahan (1991)
Newcastle upon Tyne

Purpose
Descriptive

Design
Study type:
Data type: Qualitative and quantitative
Data collection method: Closed interview schedule; focus groups
Sample type: 'Snowball'
Sample size: Interviews:
26 Bangladeshi women focus groups:
16 Bangladeshi women
Response rate:
Date study carried out:

Comments
Mean age of mothers: 29.6 (range 19–43 years)
Average time lived in UK 6.4 (range 1–15 years)

Shaukat, de Bono and Jones (1994)
Leicester

Purpose
Explanatory (observational)

Design
Study type: See below
Data type: Quantitative
Data collection method: Interview; anthropometrics blood profile
Sample type: Patient series,* and sons
Sample size: 102 'Indian origin' men, 89 sons; 102 European men, 82 sons
Response rate:†
Date study carried out: July 1992–August 1993

Comments
Interview structure not described.
Not clear if 'Indian origin' means migrant; ethnicity (Gujarati or Punjabi) 'established by grandparental route' (p. 319)
Sons were 'healthy' aged 15–30
*102 of 109 consecutive patients for angiography, matched for age and symptom duration with 102 Europeans.
†6 'Indian' sons and 4 'European' sons declined to take part

Shaunak et al. (1985)
London

Purpose
Descriptive

Design
Study type:
Data type: Quantitative
Data collection method: Administered questionnaire blood samples
Sample type: Opportunistic
Sample size: 60 Hindu couples
48 'white controls' (p.1166)
Response rate: 'About 80% of all couples present' (p. 1166)
Date study carried out: Late spring, no year given

Comments
Questionnaire was 'preset' and included a 'simple diet history' (p. 1166)
Hindu couples volunteered at social meetings of local Punjabi/Gujarati associations
White 'controls' were volunteers on staff at St George's Hospital.
Hindu couples age range: 21–75 years
White controls age range 18–62

Sheikh and Thomas (1994b)
Harrow, London

Purpose
Descriptive

Design
Study type:
Data type: Quantitative*
 Data collection method: Self-complete questionnaire; food diary
Sample type: Quota
Sample size: Unclear†
Response rate: 242/700 diaries
156/700 questionnaires
Date study carried out:

Comments
*Not clear if qualitative element although questions on food choice were open-ended. The structure of questionnaire is not described; food intake not apparently weighed
†242 diaries and 156 questionnaires – does not specify from which groups they came
Age range 12–16; 79% S. Asians were UK-born. Asian sub-groups not specified, but likely to be Hindu in this location

---

Shelley et al. (1991b)
County Kilkenny, Republic of Ireland

Purpose
Explanatory (observational)

Design
Study type: Cross-sectional
Data type: Quantitative
Data collection method: Administered questionnaire, physical measures
Sample type: Random
Sample size: 415 men, 369 women
Response rate:
Date study carried out: 1985

Comments
Serum cholesterol measured using CHOD-PAP enzymatic colorimetric method of Boehringer Mannheim. Sample aged 35–64

Sher et al. (1993)
City of Leicester

Purpose
Explanatory (observational)

Design
Study type: Retrospective
Data type: Quantitative
Data collection method: *
Sample type: Patient series
Sample size: 106 patients with coeliac disease†
Response rate: Not appropriate
Date study carried out: Diagnoses made 1975–1989

Comments
*Comprehensive list of patients with possible coeliac disease made up from hospital records, GPs (via questionnaire), The Coeliac Society (contacted members) and cross-matched with data from the two sources
†86 'European', 20 'Asian' (p. 178)

Silman et al. (1985)
Tower Hamlets, East London

Purpose
Comparative descriptive

Design
Study type:
Data type: Quantitative
 Data collection method: 'Administered' interview;* 1-day dietary observations†
Sample type: Patient series;* non-random quota for investigating diet
Sample size: Bangladeshi men: 116
Caucasian men: 211
Response rate: Bangladeshi: 50.1%
Caucasian: 58.1%
Date study carried out:

Comments
24-hour recall/diet interview considered 'inappropriate' so 12 subjects visited for a single day – weighing of raw ingredients/final portion, and cooking methods observed
Aged 35–69
*Structure not described
†Drawn from age–sex register of local general practice participating in a heart disease prevention programme. All Caucasian and Bangladeshi men aged 35–69 invited to attend for screening

---

Singleton and Tucker (1978)

Purpose
Explanatory (observational)

Design
Study type: Cross-sectional
Data type: Quantitative
Data collection method: See below
Sample type: Random, of birth registers of two health clinics
Sample size: 20 aged 18 months*
18 aged 6 months*
Response rate: 84%
Date study carried out: Second week of May 1977

Comments
Families visited twice, usually 2 days apart for quantitative recall of previous day's intake. Parents also asked about child's dietary history and feeding patterns
Vitamin D. intake from dried milks/cereals calculated from manufacturer's information
82% of sample Punjabi, mostly Sikh
*Equal numbers of each sex

Smith et al. (1993)
Bradford (two factories)

Purpose
Descriptive

Design
Study type:

Data type: Quantitative
Data collection method: Food frequency questionnaire; 3-day diet diary*
Sample type: Opportunistic†
Sample size: 126 S. Asians (78 Muslim, 44 Hindu); 160 Caucasian
Response rate: Initial: factory A 73.7%
factory B 76.2%
Caucasian v. Asian: (83.4% v. 70.6%)
Date study carried out:

Comments
†Researchers thought random sampling would 'lead to suspicion and a poor response rate' (p. 324) so men were recruited by offering 'risk assessment for heart disease'; those responding were entered into the study
*Subjects asked to include brand names and estimate portion size using household measures or weights from packets. Subjects re-interviewed by same dietitians who used food models/household measures to obtain a greater degree of accuracy in portion estimation

Solanki *et al.* (1995)
Birmingham

Purpose
Explanatory (observational)

Design
Study type: Cross-sectional
Data type: Quantitative
Data collection method: Questionnaire,* physical measures, blood samples
Sample type: Quota (volunteers)
Sample size: S. Asian: 41 elderly (aged over 65), 24 young white: 20 elderly, 21 young
Response rate: Not applicable
Date study carried out: Last week of March–first week of April, year unstated

Comments
Elderly S. Asians recruited from GP lists and day centres; elderly whites recruited from local church day centre; young S. Asians and white controls: hospital staff
SA elderly: 23 men, 18 women (mean age 72 (range 67–91))
SA young: 19 men, 5 women (mean age 31 (range 19–63))
White elderly: 5 men, 15 women (mean age 74 (range 67–83))
White young: 6 men, 15 women (mean age 30 (range 20–64))
*Not clear if administered or self-complete; structure not described, but topics included dietary habits

Stephens *et al.* (1982)
Rochdale

Purpose
Explanatory (experimental)

Design
Study type: Before-and-after*
Data type: Quantitative
Data collection method: 3-day and 7-day recall
Sample type: S. Asian: self-referral†

Caucasian: random
Sample size: S. Asians: 150 adults, 103 children
 Caucasian: 36 adults, 34 children
Response rate:
Date study carried out: 1980

Comments
Follow-up of dietary survey in 1970 which prompted campaign to improve vitamin D status of S. Asians
*Same population but not same individuals
†To specially arranged clinics; Caucasian children sampled from school registers, adults from electoral register

Strachan *et al.* (1995)
Wandsworth tuberculosis clinic, South London

Purpose
Explanatory (observational)

Design
Study type: Case-control
Data type: Quantitative
Data collection method: Structured questionnaire, food frequency questionnaire
Sample type: Cases: patient series controls: quota*
Sample size: Cases: 56, controls 100
Response rate: Cases: unknown; controls (initial) 23/340
Date study carried out: No earlier than 1993

Comments
*Cases: patients from TB clinic diagnosed with active TB in last 10 years; controls from randomly chosen starting points in record stack so that distribution by date of birth (within decades) matched those of cases. 30 general practices sampled. Low control response rate, so community/OP clinic controls recruited
Cases/controls (all migrant) classified by surname to S. Asian religious group
Cases: 22 male, 34 female: 33 Hindu, 20 Muslim, 3 other
Controls: 39 male, 61 female; 46 Hindu, 49 Muslim, 5 other
Born 1903–39: 20 cases, 29 controls
Born 1940–54: 14 cases, 39 controls
Born 1955–73: 22 cases, 32 controls

Tauber *et al.* (1980)
Tower Hamlets, East London

Purpose
Explanatory (experimental)

Design
Study type: Cross-sectional
Data type: Quantitative
Data collection method: *
Sample type: Opportunistic
Sample size: 133 Bengali women
Response rate:
Date study carried out:

Comments
*Identification of food items in series of pictures and line

drawings; 'correct' answer was available on back of photograph, and interviewers entered 'correct', 'wrong' or 'doubtful' on to pro forma. Interviewers were fluent in Bengali/Sylheti

Respondents included if they had not gone to school in UK, and did not work in UK as health professional, teacher or similar

Women's ages not given

Thompson and Cruickshank (1990)
North West London

Purpose
Descriptive

Design
Study type: Cross-sectional
Data type: Quantitative
Data collection method: Diet history questionnaire, validated with 5-day weighed inventory
Sample type: Random*
Sample size: 15 Gujarati women†
27 African-Caribbean women
Response rate:
Date study carried out:

Comments
Abstract only
*Forms part of a population survey
†Vegetarian

Treuherz, Cullinan and Saunders (1982)
Hackney and Tower Hamlets, East London

Purpose
Descriptive

Design
Study type:
Data type: Quantitative
Data collection method: Administered questionnaire
Sample type: *
Sample size: 3712 babies* (inc. 690 'Asian' babies)
Response rate:
Date study carried out: March 1979–February 1980

Comments
*'All but a few babies' living in Hackney and Tower Hamlets; method of contact not described
Mothers interviewed when baby 4 weeks; structure of questionnaire not described
'Entered the study' – figures for 'missing' infants added to total do not add up to 3712 in most tables – Asian not differentiated

Versi et al. (1995)
East London

Purpose
Comparative descriptive

Design
Study type: Retrospective
Data type: Quantitative
Data collection method: Review of obstetric data
Sample type: Patient series (complete)
Sample size: 'White Caucasian' 7592
Bangladeshi 6460
Response rate: Not applicable
Date study carried out: See below

Comments
Study of 16 718 pregnancies 1987–1991; comparison of age, parity, ante-natal complications, details of labour, 3rd stage complication rates, gestation, birthweights and perinatal mortality rates (based on no. of infants delivered live/stillborn after 28 weeks of gestation)
2666 Indian, Pakistani, West Indian, African and Oriental women were not considered further in this study

Viegas et al. (1982a)
Sorrento Maternity Hospital, Birmingham

Purpose
Explanatory (experimental)

Design
Study type: Controlled intervention trial
Data type: Quantitative
Data collection method:
Sample type: Patient series*
Sample size: 153 S. Asian women
Response rate:
Date study carried out: 25 April–29 October 1979

Comments
Three regimes of unselective dietary protein energy supplementation in second and third trimesters
*Booked before 20 weeks gestation and living within defined area of city of Birmingham

Viegas et al. (1982b)
Sorrento Maternity Hospital, Birmingham

Purpose
Explanatory (experimental)

Design
Study type: Controlled intervention trial
Data type: Quantitative
Data collection method:
Sample type: Patient series*
Sample size: 130 S. Asian women
Response rate:
Date study carried out: 5 November 1979–11 June 1980

Comments
Selective supplementation in third trimester only: 45 mothers nutritionally at risk at 28 weeks given 1 of 3 supplements; 83 regarded as adequately nourished also received one supplement
*Booked before 20 weeks gestation and living within defined area of city of Birmingham

Ward et al. (1988)

SSG Hospital and Kalpana Clinic, Baroda, Gujarat, India;
Northwick Park Hospital, Harrow

Purpose
Explanatory (observational)

Design
Study type: Longitudinal
Data type: Quantitative
Data collection method: 7-day dietary recall*
Sample type: Patient series†
Sample size: Baroda: 73 Gujarati women
Harrow: 92 Indian women
Response rate:
Date study carried out:

Comments
*Information on dietary, social and ethnic origins collected at 28 weeks gestation in manner comparable to previous study and results from Baroda compared to previous study results (Campbell-Brown et al., 1995). Birthweight of 31 Baroda babies available.
†Healthy pregnant women recruited from two outpatient clinics
Baroda: 53 vegetarian, 20 non-vegetarian
Harrow: 59 vegetarian, 33 non-vegetarian

Wardle, Wrightson and Gibson (1996)

South London

Purpose
Comparative descriptive

Design
Study type: Quantitative
Data collection method:*
Sample type: Stratified random†
Sample size: 49 S. Asian (no sub-groups) mothers and children
63 European mothers and children
Response rate: c. 50% across 7 practices
Date study carried out:

Comments
*No description of data collection apart from anthropometric methods (minimal) and abdominal fatness indices
†Randomly selected families with children in designated age range from 7 GP registers in S. London, including 3 known to include a high proportion of S. Asians
Women's age: S. Asian 37.63 +/- 5.4; European 40.32 +/- 4.3; Children's age: S. Asians 10.61 +/- 1.2; European 10.72 +/– 0.87

Warrington and Storey (1988a)

Rochdale

Purpose
Explanatory (observational)

Design
Study type: Longitudinal
Data type: Quantitative
Data collection method: 3-day weighed intake
Sample type: Patient series*
Sample size: S. Asian: 28 male, 27 female†
Caucasian: 28 male, 27 female
Response rate:
Date study carried out:

Comments
*Infants all first-born and selected from concurrent births with exclusion of caesarian births; severe illness in neonatal period; birthweight below 1000 g; congenital abnormalities; neurological damage
Growth of two groups compared in first two years
†Matched with Caucasian for sex and socioeconomic status (except 2 male Asians and four female Caucasians)

Warrington and Storey (1988b)

Rochdale

Purpose
Explanatory (observational)

Design
Study type: Longitudinal
Data type: Quantitative
Data collection method: 3-day weighed intake*
Sample type: Patient series
Sample size: S. Asian: 28 male, 27 female
Caucasian: 28 male, 27 female
Response rate:
Date study carried out:

Comments
See above for details of study design
*Breast milk intakes measured by test-weighing method, and vitamin supplements were included in the data. Intakes were estimated at 3, 6, 9, 12, 24 months of age

Wharton, Eaton and Wharton (1984)

Sorrento Maternity Hospital, Birmingham

Purpose
Descriptive

Design
Study type:
Data type: Quantitative
Data collection method: Weighed 3-day intake, and 24-hour recall
Sample type: Patient series
Sample size: 90 Pakistani Muslim
36 Sikh; 29 Hindu;
10 Bangladeshi Muslim
Response rate:
Date study carried out: January–November, year unstated

Comments
Style of reporting makes ascertainment of sample size and

methodology problematic

3 weekday weighed intakes at 18, 23, 28, 33, 38 weeks (combined for analysis because of small numbers in places) of every 5th women taking part in supplement trial (see Viegas *et al.*, 1982a and b)

Intakes of other women recalled once in each trimester at 23 and 33 weeks

†Booked before 20 weeks gestation and living within defined area of city of Birmingham

Williams, Sahota and Fairpo (1989)

Inner city Leeds

Purpose
Descriptive

Design
Study type:
Data type: Quantitative
Data collection method: Administered 'structured' interview
Sample type: S. Asian† infants: quota 'white' infants: random
Sample size: S. Asian: 184
White: 127
Response rate:
Date study carried out:

Comments
Home-based interview conducted by multi-lingual female interpreter; 'white' female interviewer for 'white' families
White infants selected from birth register
All infants aged 6–24 months – balance of ages similar between S. Asian and white. In both groups, families excluded if 'handicapping problems' or infant spent considerable time away from home each day, e.g. at nursery
†50 Bangladeshi (Sylhet), 55 Pakistani (Mirpur), 49 Punjabi Sikh, 28 Gujarati. Majority of families resident in UK for less than 15 years

Williams, Bhopal and Hunt (1993)

Glasgow

Purpose
Explanatory (observational)

Design
Study type: Cross-sectional
Data type: Quantitative
Data collection method: Administered, closed interview schedule*
Sample type: Two-stage stratified random cluster
Sample size: S. Asian: 159, general population: 319
Response rate: S. Asian 73.6%, general population: –
Date study carried out: 1987

Comments
Subsample of the West of Scotland Twenty-07 Study: a population-based, cross-sectional and cohort studies of lifestyle and health in the West of Scotland
S. Asians aged 30–40, mean age 35; general population aged 35
*Plus anthropometrics, lung function, medical history

Williams, Bhopal and Hunt (1994)

Glasgow

Purpose
Explanatory (observational)

Design
Study type: Cross-sectional
Data type: Quantitative
Data collection method: Administered, closed interview schedule
Sample type: Two-stage stratified random cluster
Sample size: S. Asian: 173, general population: 344
Response rate: S. Asian 80.5%, general population: –
Date study carried out: 1987

Comments
Included dietary questions concerning broad patterns of food choice and frequency of consumption, modelled on Health and Lifestyle Survey (1987) with appropriate additions for South Asians
Sub-sample of the West of Scotland Twenty-07 Study: a population-based, cross-sectional and cohort studies of lifestyle and health in the West of Scotland
S. Asians: 86% Punjabi speakers, 89% born in Indian subcontinent; all arrived in UK 1950–1986
S. Asians aged 30–40, mean age 35; general population aged 35

Woollett *et al.* (1995)

Newham, East London

Purpose
Explanatory (observational)

Design
Study type: Cross-sectional
Data type: Quantitative/qualitative (subset of South Asian)
Data collection method: Structured interview, plus tape-recorded open questions
Sample type: Patient series (ante-natal)
Sample size: South Asian: 100
non-South Asian: 43
Response rate:*
Date study carried out:

Comments
Pregnant women who had at least one child.
32 qualitative interviews of S. Asians conducted in respondents' homes – desire to be interviewed at home rather than in ante-natal clinic seems to have determined whether interviewed qualitatively as well as quantitatively. Interviewer spoke fluent English, Hindi, Punjabi and Urdu
S. Asian: 47% Muslim, 36% Hindu, 17% Sikh
Non-S. Asian: 98% Christian, 2% Muslim
Non-S. Asian: 20 'white', 3 Irish, 8 African, 12 Caribbean – 10 non-S. Asian not born in UK
S. Asian: mean age 27 years, range 20–41
Non-S. Asian: mean age 26.5, range 18–37
*3 refusals, 2 not at home, 10 interviews not completed at clinic for lack of time – total approached not known

Wright (1995)

Northern Ireland

Purpose

Explanatory (observational)

Design

Study type: Case-control
Data type: Quantitative
Data collection method: 7-day weighed dietary intake;
interview schedule
Sample type: Cases: patient series controls
Sample size: Cases: 15
controls 15

Response rate:
Date study carried out:

Comments

Cases had recently had a baby or a terminated pregnancy
affected by neural tube defect; controls had recently had a
normal baby
20 ml blood collected on completion of weighed intake;
height and weight noted
Interview (structure not given) included questions on food
habits and preferences, smoking/alcohol, nutrition education,
medical and obstetric history
Controls selected by each subject's GP, matching for age
+/– 5 years, parity, social class based on occupation of head
of household and length of time since delivery
Cases/controls were aged 20–49

Appendix B. Ethnic group classifications used in the 1991 Census

Categories used in the ethnic group question

Respondents were asked to describe their ethnic group by ticking the relevant box from a set of pre-defined categories: White, Black – Caribbean, Black – African, Indian, Pakistani, Bangladeshi and Chinese. If none of these was appropriate, respondents were asked to indicate either 'Black – Other' or 'Any other ethnic group' and then describe their ethnic origin in the free text fields provided. These answers were then assigned to one of the following 35 codes:

Code	Category
0	White
1	Black – Caribbean
2	Black – African
3	Indian
4	Pakistani
5	Bangladeshi
6	Chinese

Black – Other: non-mixed origin

7	British
8	Caribbean Island, West Indies or Guyana
9	North African, Arab or Iranian
10	Other African countries
11	East African Asian or Indo-Caribbean
12	Indian sub-continent
13	Other Asian
14	Other answers

Black – Other: mixed origin

15	Black/White
16	Asian/White
17	Other mixed

Other ethnic group: non-mixed origin

18	British – minority ethnic indicated
19	British – no minority ethnic indicated
20	Caribbean Island, West Indies or Guyana
21	North African, Arab or Iranian
22	East African
24	Indian sub-continent
25	Other Asian
26	Irish
27	Greek (including Greek Cypriot)
28	Turkish (including Turkish Cypriot)

| 29 | Other Europeans |
| 30 | Other answers |

Other ethnic group: mixed origin

31	Black/White
32	Asian/White
33	Mixed White
34	Other mixed

10-category output classification

White	0 26–29 33
Black – Caribbean	1 8 20
Black – African	2 10 22
Black – Other	7 14 15 17
Indian	3
Pakistani	4
Bangladeshi	5
Chinese	6
Other groups – Asian	11–13 23–25
– Other	9 16 18 19 21 30–32 34

Source: Aspinall, 1996, pp. 11–12

Appendix C. Databases and keywords

Databases searched
SHARE (Race and Ethnicity), Kings Fund, London (1991–1996)
Centre for Research in Ethnic Relations (online), University of Warwick (1987–1996)
Ethnic Minorities Health (1990–1996)
Ethnic Health Bibliography (selected bibliography published in 1993, covers references from 1971)
DHSS Database (1980–1996)
Medline (1980–1996)
BIDS (Embase) (1981–1996)
BIDS (Social Sciences Citation Index) (1981–1996)
Applied Social Sciences Index & Abstracts (ASSIA) (1981–1996)
Accompline (for 'grey' literature) (1980–1996)
CRIB (Current Research in Britain)
Reuters (newspaper reports) (1980–1996)
The Magazine Index (for 'popular' as opposed to academic articles) (1980–1996)

Keywords

ethnic	weight	intake
South Asian	anthropometrics	nutrition
Indian sub-continent	coronary	nutrient
Indian	ischaemic	triglycerides
Pakistani	cardiovascular	cholesterol
Bangladeshi	stroke	fat
Punjabi	blood pressure	carbohydrate
Gujarati	tuberculosis	protein
Sikh	diabetes	vitamin
Muslim	metabolic	iron
Moslem	disturbances	fruit
Hindu	insulin	vegetables
Irish	glucose	meat
Ireland	cancer	vegetarian
	rickets	vegan
health status	osteomalacia	snack
mortality	growth	meal
morbidity	pregnancy	cuisine
obesity	ante-natal	hospitality
adipose	birthweight	feast
body	breast-feeding	fasting
waist	weaning	drug
hip	eat	alcohol
stature	food	parenting
height	diet	child-rearing

single parent
family
dependants
housing
household
extended
homeless
deprivation

poverty
employment
unemployment
income
social class
socioeconomic
economic
disadvantage

qualifications
education
ethnic business
market change
food marketing
beliefs

Appendix D. Example of pro forma for searching BIDS databases

BIDS IS/EMBASE (circle) 1984–1986

Ethnicity	South Asian	Indian sub-continent	Indian	Muslim	Hindu	Irish	Ireland
health status							
mortality							
morbidity							
obesity							
adipose							
body							
waist							
hip							
stature							
height							
weight							
anthropometrics							
coronary							
ischaemic							
cardiovascular							
stroke							
blood pressure							
tuberculosis							
diabetes							
metabolic disturbances							
insulin							
glucose							
cancer							
rickets							
osteomalacia							
growth							
pregnancy							
ante-natal							
birthweight							
breast-feeding							
weaning							
eat							
food							

Ethnicity	South Asian	Indian sub-continent	Indian	Muslim	Hindu	Irish	Ireland
diet							
intake							
nutrition							
nutrient							
triglycerides							
cholesterol							
fat							
carbohydrate							
protein							
vitamin							
iron							
fruit							
vegetables							
meat							
vegetarian							
vegan							
snack							
meal							
cuisine							
hospitality							
feast							
fasting							
drug							
alcohol							
parenting							
child-rearing							
single parent							
family							
dependants							
housing							
household							
extended							
homeless							
deprivation							
poverty							
employment							
unemployment							
income							
social class							

Ethnicity	South Asian	Indian sub-continent	Indian	Muslim	Hindu	Irish	Ireland
socioeconomic							
economic							
disadvantage							
qualifications							
education							
ethnic business							
market change							
food marketing							
beliefs							

	Pakistani	Punjabi	Bangladeshi	Gujarati	Sikh

Appendix E. Report tables

Table 1. Mean daily intake of energy, protein, vitamin D and iron in pregnant South Asian women

	Method of dietary data collection	Energy (kcal) (mean and range/SD)	Protein (g) (mean and range/SD)	Vitamin D μg (mean and range/SD)	Iron (mg) (mean and range/SD)
COMA recommendation (Department of Health, 1991)		1940 (+ 200 in 3rd trimester)	51	10.00	12
Wharton, Eaton and Wharton, 1984	Weighed and recall				
Pakistani Muslim (n = 90)		1589 (488–4316)	56 (16–210)	0.90 (0–4.6)	11 (3–32)
Bangladeshi Muslim (n = 10)		1555 (627–1955)	59 (16–118)	1.51 (0.7–3.6)	9 (4–15)
Sikh (n = 36)		1800 (940–3872)	53 (24–106)	0.98 (0.2–3.4)	12 (5–28)
Hindu (n = 29)		1790 (1080–2981)	60 (29–117)	1.30 (0.1–4.9)	10 (6–17)
Abraham et al., 1985 South Asians (sub-groups combined (n = 813)	7-day recall	2010 (+/- 532)			
Hindu vegetarians* (n = 450)			57.2 (+/-15.8)		
Hindu non-vegetarians (n = 225)			66.6 (+/-17.2)		
Muslim non-vegetarians (n = 138)			65.9 (+/-19.9)		
Abraham et al., 1987	7-day recall				
Hindu vegetarians* (n = 450)				1.04 (+/- 0.91)	10.20 (+/- 3.25)
Hindu non-vegetarians (n = 225)				1.65 (+/-1.82)	10.86 (+/- 3.21)
Muslim non-vegetarians (n = 138)				1.95 (+/- 2.31)	11.28 (+/- 3/49)
Henriksen et al., 1995 Pakistani (n = 58)	Diet history (1 month)			2.2 (1.5–3.4)	
Brunvald et al., 1995 Pakistani (n = 38)	Diet history (1 month)				10.9 (10.0–11.8)

*Three categories of varying strictness combined in original paper

Table 2. Mean per cent total energy intake from fat in South Asians

Respondents	Sample size	Mean % total energy intake from fat	Authors
Gujarati women (pregnant)	813	44	Abraham et al., 1985
Bangladeshi men	12	60	Silman et al., 1985
Gujarati (mainly) men and women	184	39	McKeigue et al., 1985
Gujarati (mainly) diabetic patients	48	46	Peterson et al., 1986
Indian men	20	38	Miller et al., 1988
Punjabi Sikh and Muslim women	104	40	Henderson et al., 1990
Muslim* men	78	39	Smith et al., 1993
Hindu* men	44	42	Smith et al., 1993
Punjabi men	92	36	Sevak, McKeigue and Marmot, 1994
Punjabi women, migrant, Muslim (mainly)	35	42	Anderson et al., 1995
Punjabi women, British-born, Muslim (mainly)	37	40	Anderson et al., 1995
Punjabi Sikh and Muslim women†	10	36	Anderson and Lean, 1995
Indian-descent women (pre-menopausal, vegetarian)	22	38	Reddy and Sanders, 1992
Gujarati women (vegetarian)	15	40	Thompson and Cruickshank, 1990

*Country of origin not given
†Follow-up of women from Henderson et al., 1990

Table 3. Mean waist/hip ratio and body mass index of South Asians in Britain

Sample	Age	Sample size	Mean waist/hip ratio	Mean body mass index	Author
Women (migrant), mainly Punjabi, Glasgow	30–40	159	0.84 (SD 0.06)	27.0 (SD 6.3)	Williams, Bhopal and Hunt, 1993
Men (migrant), mainly Punjabi, Glasgow	30–40	(Total)	0.94 (SD 0.05)	25.4 (SD 3.8)	
Women (migrant), mainly Punjabi, Glasgow	20–40	62	0.88 (SD 0.01)	267.0 (SD 0.55)	Bush et al., 1995
Women (British-born), mainly Punjabi, Glasgow	20–40	56	0.84 (SD 0.01)	25.7 (SD 0.77)	Bush et al., 1995
Women (migrant), 52% Sikh, West London	40–69	291	0.85 (0.84–0.86)	27.0 (26.5–27.5)	McKeigue, Shah and Marmot, 1991
Men (migrant), 52% Sikh, West London	40–69	1421	0.98 (0.97–0.98)	25.7 (25.5–25.8)	McKeigue, Shah and Marmot, 1991
Men (not stated), 52% Sikh, Bradford	20–65	110	0.92 (0.91–0.94)	23.8 (23.2–24.4)	Knight et al., 1992
Male (migrant), Pakistani, Peterborough	20 and over	100	–	25.2 (SD 4.13)	Bose, 1995
Female (British-born), not differentiated, London	19	34	1.11* (SE 0.01)	22.1 (SE 0.06)	Gishen, Hogh and Stock, 1995
Male (British-born), not differentiated, London	19	60	1.19* (SE 0.01)	23.6 (SE 0.05)	Gishen, Hogh and Stock, 1995
Female, † not differentiated, Oxford	20–23	40	0.79 (0.78–0.81)	22.0 (21.2–22.7)	Potts and Simmons, 1994
Male,† not differentiated, Oxford	20–23	40	0.87 (0.85–0.89)	21.3 (20.4–22.1)	
Indian-descent women (vegetarian)	Pre-menopausal	22	0.77 (SE 0.014)	25.1 (SE 0.98)	Reddy and Sanders, 1992

*Conicity index (w/0.109 square root (W/H))

†93% total sample (male and female) British-born, 7% lived in UK for minimum of 14 years

Table 4. Body mass index (BMI) and total dietary energy intake with percentage of energy contributed by macronutrients

	African-Caribbean men n = 85	NDNS* White men n = 273	African-Caribbean women n = 125	NDNS* White women n = 283
Mean age (years)	57.1	–	51.2	–
CI† (= range)	54–60	50–64†	49–54	50–64†
Mean BMI kg/m²	27.0	25.9	28.7	26.2
CI	26.3–27.7	25.5–26.3	27.7–29.8	25.5–26.9
Energy (kcal)	2334	2380	1926	1610
CI	2142–2526	2319–2441	1802–2051	1564–1656
(kJoules)	9765	9958	8058	6736
CI	8962–10 569	9703–10 213	7540–8581	6544–6929
% Carbohydrate	48.9	41.4	51.0	42.3
CI	47.2–50.5	40.6–42.2	49.9–52.1	41.9–42.7
% Alcohol	n = 77		n = 103	
(drinkers only)	3.9	8.1	1.6	3.5
CI	3.0–4.9	7.1–9.1	1.3–1.9	2.9–4.1
% Fat	32.0	37.6	32.6	39.5
CI	30.9–33.1	37–38.2	31.7–33.5	38.9–40
% Saturated fat	11.5	16.1	11.9	17.1
CI	10.3–12.7	15.7–16.5	10.7–13.0	17.3–17.5
% Protein	14.9	14.7	14.7	16.1
% CI	14.5–15.3	14.4–15.0	14.3–15.1	15.7–16.5

kcal to kJoules: x 4.184

*National Diet and Nutritional Survey of British Adults
†CI = 95% confidence intervals

Table 5. Mean daily intakes of energy, fat, fibre and iron of men in the Republic of Ireland, Northern Ireland and Britain

	Energy (k/cal day)		Fat (g/day)		Fat (% of energy)*		Fibre (g/day)		Iron (mg/day)	
	Mean	*SD*	*Mean*	*SD*	*Mean*	*SD*	*Mean*	*SD*	*Mean*	*SD*
Republic†										
18–25 (*n* = 51)	3273	1070	133.0	58.00	35.5	6.7	22.1	12.2	15.4	4.9
25–40 (*n* = 85)	3035	781	123.0	39.00	36.2	5.8	20.3	7.9	15.0	4.0
40–60 (*n* = 87)	2526	757	98.0	39.00	34.3	6.3	19.6	8.8	13.1	4.8
60+ (*n* = 82)	2262	739	85.0	35.00	33.4	6.0	20.1	10.4	11.2	4.1
Northern Ireland										
	Mean	*SD*	*Mean*	*SD*	*Mean*	*SD*	*Mean*	*SD*	*Mean*	*SD*
16–29 (*n* = 105)	2557	605	111.4	29.80	39.2	–	20.5	7.19	13.3	6.36
30–39 (*n* = 64)	2671	541	112.7	30.11	37.8	–	22.2	8.17	14.2	4.43
40–49 (*n* = 51)	2417	567	103.3	24.38	38.8	–	19.4	7.78	12.8	4.88
50–64 (*n* = 38)	2343	554	102.3	33.56	38.9	–	21.4	7.90	14.9	6.06
All ages (*n* = 258)	2526	583	108.8	29.63	38.7	–	20.8	7.68	13.6	5.63
Britain										
	Mean	*SE*	*Mean*	*SE*	*Mean*	*SE*	*Mean*	*SE*	*Mean*	*SE*
16–24 (*n* = 214)	2460	47	103.5	2.14	37.9	0.36	23.9	0.56	13.0	0.35
25–34 (*n* = 254)	2440	38	103.1	1.79	37.9	0.32	24.5	0.56	14.1	0.37
35–49 (*n* = 346)	2500	32	103.3	1.51	37.1	0.28	25.8	0.50	14.5	0.32
50–64 (*n* = 273)	2380	31	99.4	1.51	37.6	0.32	24.8	0.53	14.1	0.30
All ages (*n* = 1087)	2450	18	102.3	0.85	37.6	0.16	24.9	0.27	14.0	0.17
COMA/NACNE‡										
15–18	2755				33.0		30.0‡		11.3	
19–50	2550				33.0		30.0‡		8.7	
50+									8.7	

Sources: Barker *et al.*, 1989; Gregory *et al.*, 1990; Irish Nutrition and Dietetic Institute, 1990

*As % contribution to total energy intake (i.e. including alcohol)
†Summary figures for 'all ages' not provided
‡ See final paragraph, page 68

Table 6. Mean daily intakes of energy, fat, fibre and iron of women in the Republic of Ireland, Northern Ireland and Britain

	Energy (k/cal day)		Fat (g/day)		Fat (% of energy)*		Fibre (g/day)		Iron (mg/day)	
*Republic***	*Mean*	*SD*	*Mean*	*SD*	*Mean*	*SD*	*Mean*	*SD*	*Mean*	*SD*
18–25 (*n* =54)	2048	878	85.0	46	36.4	6.5	15.6	7.0	10.8	4.9
25–40 (*n* =122)	1842	701	73.0	31	35.3	6.2	16.5	7.9	10.8	4.4
40–60 (*n* =111)	1748	600	70.0	32	34.9	6.9	16.7	8.5	10.0	3.7
60+ (*n* =84)	1710	592	65.0	27	33.8	6.1	18.2	9.1	9.8	3.4
Northern Ireland	*Mean*	*SD*	*Mean*	*SD*	*Mean*	*SD*	*Mean*	*SD*	*Mean*	*SD*
16–29 (*n* =110)	1816	443	80.8	23.69	39.7	–	16.4	5.58	10.6	5.59
30–39 (*n* =90)	1721	446	76.0	22.56	39.6	–	16.2	6.44	10.5	4.77
40–49 (*n* =70)	1673	482	73.4	26.57	38.9	–	16.6	6.68	10.8	4.43
50–64 (*n* =64)	1499	325	68.0	19.03	40.5	–	14.5	4.77	9.1	2.66
All ages (*n* =334)	1670	445	75.5	23.57	39.6	–	16.0	5.95	10.3	4.70
Britain	*Mean*	*SE*	*Mean*	*SE*	*Mean*	*SE*	*Mean*	*SE*	*Mean*	*SE*
16–24 (*n* =189)	1700	32	73.6	1.61	38.7	0.33	17.4	0.47	11.8	0.95
25–34 (*n* =253)	1670	29	73.6	1.51	39.4	0.33	18.2	0.41	11.1	0.42
35–49 (*n* =385)	1730	23	75.5	1.19	39.0	0.29	18.9	0.34	12.9	0.69
50–64 (*n* =283)	1610	23	70.9	1.21	39.5	0.29	19.3	0.38	12.9	0.78
All ages (*n* =1110)	1680	13	73.5	0.68	39.2	0.16	18.6	0.20	12.3	0.36
COMA/NACNE†										
15–18	2110				33.0		30.0‡		14.8	
19–50	1940				33.0		30.0‡		14.8†	
50+	1900								8.7	

Sources: Barker *et al.*, 1989; Gregory *et al.*, 1990; Irish Nutrition and Dietetic Institute, 1990

*As % contribution to total energy intake (i.e. including alcohol)
**Summary figures for 'all ages' not provided
†Iron supplement required for women with high menstrual losses
‡See final paragraph, page 68

Table 7. Distribution of body mass index (W/H2) of men and women in the Republic of Ireland and Northern Ireland

Kilkenny Health Project (% by sex)

	Males			Females		
	BMI range	Number	%	BMI range	Number	%
Underweight	< 20.1	9	2.2	< 18.7	7	1.9
Acceptable	20.1–25.0	137	33.0	18.7–23.8	126	34.2
Overweight	25.1–29.9	212	51.1	23.9–28.5	165	44.7
Obese	30.0*	57	13.7	28.6*	71	19.2

*Greater than or equal to
Source: Shelley *et al.*, 1991b

Northern Ireland (% by age and sex)

Males	BMI range	16–29	30–39	40–49	50–64
Underweight	< 20.0	17.3	2.9	1.9	2.4
Acceptable	20.1–25.0	55.8	38.2	36.5	36.6
Overweight	25.1–29.9	24.0	47.1	46.1	53.7
Obese	> 30.0	2.9	11.8	15.4	7.3
Number		104	68	52	41

Females	BMI range	16–29	30–39	40–49	50–64
	< 18.6	6.5	5.6	1.4	2.8
	18.7–23.8	57.9	47.7	41.7	26.4
	23.9–28.5	28.0	35.5	36.1	45.8
	> 28.6	7.5	12.2	20.8	25.0
Number		107	90	72	72

Source: Barker *et al.*, 1989

Great Britain (cumulative % by age and sex)

Males	BMI*	16–24	25–34	35–49	50–64
	20 or less	15	4	4	5
	25 or less	79	64	48	38
	30 or less	97	94	89	91
Number		222	269	369	298

Females	BMI*	16–24	25–34	35–49	50–64
	20 or less	25	17	8	5
	25 or less	77	73	60	54
	30 or less	94	89	90	82
Number		193	261	402	305

Source: Gregory *et al.*, 1990

*20 or less = underweight, over 20 to 25 = average, over 25 to 30 = overweight, over 30 = obese (Gregory *et al.*, 1990, p. 230)

Table 8. Body mass index (W/H2) of men and women in the Republic of Ireland, Northern Ireland and Britain

	Males			Females		
Kilkenny Health Project	No.	Mean	SD	No.	Mean	SD
35–44	178	25.9	–	158	24.7	–
45-54	118	26.8	–	114	26.2	–
55-64	119	26.7	–	97	25.9	–
Total	415	26.4	–	369	25.5	–
Northern Ireland	No.	Mean	SD	No.	Mean	SD
16–29	104	23.5	3.28	107	23.0	3.28
30–39	68	25.8	3.51	90	24.2	4.11
40–49	52	26.0	3.52	72	25.6	4.40
50–64	41	25.7	2.82	72	26.3	4.32
Total	265	24.9	3.49	341	24.6	4.17
Great Britain	No.	Mean	SE	No.	Mean	SE
16–24	222	22.9	0.22	193	22.9	0.35
25–34	269	24.6	0.20	261	23.9	0.33
35–49	369	25.6	0.19	402	24.8	0.21
50–64	298	25.9	0.19	305	26.2	0.33
Total	1158	24.9	0.11	1161	24.6	0.15

Sources: Shelley et al., 1991b; Barker et al., 1989; Gregory et al., 1990

Table 9. Economic characteristics of South Asians, African-Caribbeans, Irish and the ethnic majority ('white') in Britain

	Indian		Pakistani		Bangladeshi		African-Caribbean		Irish-born		'White'	
	Male	Female	Male	Female	Male	Female	Male	Female	Male	Female	Male	Female
Aged 16–59/64:												
economic activity rate	82.3	60.4	75.7	28.3	74.3	22.2	80.1	66.9	85.6	69.6	87.0	68.3
unemployment rate	13.4	12.7	28.5	29.6	30.9	34.5	23.8	13.5	15.0	7.0	10.7	6.3
Economically inactive aged 16+												
inactivity rate	21.9	44.6	26.7	22.9	27.6	78.2	19.9	33.1	29.9	50.1	26.9	50.3
full-time students (%)	46.6	19.5	48.3	12.9	44.9	14.5	21.9	16.3	4.5	2.5	13.5	6.7
permanently sick (%)	21.6	10.0	28.9	4.8	31.5	2.8	27.4	14.9	26.1	8.8	18.5	6.6
retired (%)	26.4	12.7	14.6	3.6	13.9	2.6	43.0	25.8	65.9	46.9	65.2	42.9
other inactive (%)	5.4	57.8	8.2	78.8	9.8	80.0	7.8	42.9	3.5	41.8	2.7	43.9
Self-employed (%)	25.3	12.7	26.6	15.6	20.9	8.8	10.2	1.9	20.1	5.3	17.6	6.6

Source: Owen, 1994a; 1995 (based on 1991 Census Local Base Statistics)

Table 10. Social class of South Asians, African-Caribbeans, Irish and the ethnic majority ('white') in Britain

Social class	Indian		Pakistani		Bangladeshi		African-Caribbean		Irish-born		'White'	
	Male	Female	Male	Female	Male	Female	Male	Female	Male	Female	Male	Female
I	11.4	4.4	5.9	2.7	5.2	1.8	2.4	1.0	6.9	2.6	6.7	1.7
II	27.2	20.9	20.3	22.3	8.5	22.9	14.2	30.3	23.3	33.2	27.6	25.9
III (non-manual)	14.4	34.9	13.5	34.2	12.9	35.8	12.2	33.7	7.7	26.8	11.3	39.0
III (manual)	23.8	6.4	29.9	6.5	31.5	6.4	38.9	6.9	34.3	6.3	32.4	7.6
IV	18.1	29.2	24.1	31.7	35.0	26.6	23.6	19.5	16.9	18.5	16.3	17.8
V	4.0	4.1	6.3	2.6	6.8	6.4	8.7	8.5	10.9	12.6	5.7	8.0

Source: Owen, 1994a; Peach, 1996 (based on 1991 Census Local Base Statistics and 2 per cent SARs)

Table 11. Family composition and marital status of South Asians, African-Caribbeans, Irish and the ethnic majority ('white') in Britain

	Indian		Pakistani		Bangladeshi		African-Caribbean		Irish-born	'White'	
All families (10% sample)	21 364		9758		2942		14 098		43 064	1 462 155	
married couple families with one or more dependent children	58.8		68.0		75.1		20.3		26.8	25.0	
cohabiting couple familes with one or more dependent children	0.5		0.5		0.4		5.2		1.9	2.5	
lone parent families with one or more dependent children	5.4		9.4		11.3		30.8		8.0	7.8	
Percentage aged 16 and over:	M	F	M	F	M	F	M	F		M	F
single	27.0	21.2	29.2	21.9	32.7	21.5	47.2	50.0		29.5	22.6
married	69.6	68.3	68.7	71.3	66.2	71.4	42.2	35.2		61.0	56.1
widowed	1.6	7.6	0.9	4.7	0.4	5.9	2.0	4.2		3.9	14.5
divorced	1.9	2.9	1.3	2.1	0.7	1.2	8.6	10.7		5.5	6.8

	N Ireland (M)	N Ireland (F)	Republic (M)	Republic (F)
Percentage aged 16 and over:				
single	29.4	25.8	25.0	19.2
married	53.6	48.7	58.0	53.0
widowed	3.9	12.4	5.5	16.2
divorced	13.1	13.1	11.5	11.6

Source: Owen, 1994a; 1994b; 1995, based on 1991 Census local base statistics, OPCS/General Register for Scotland (1994) *1991 Census: Ethnic group and country of birth: Great Britain.*

Table 12. Description of traditional foods eaten by African-Caribbeans

Food	Description
Hard dough	Dense white bread, usually unsliced loaf
Bun	Sweet flavoured bread, usually eaten with sliced hard cheese, e.g. cheddar
Jamaican crackers	Similar to cream crackers but round and smaller, made with white flour
Cornmeal porridge	Made with hot milk and cornmeal flour (condensed milk may be added), flavoured with fresh nutmeg, salt, sugar and vanilla
Callaloo	Green leaves like spinach, available tinned (usually in brine) or fresh, often cooked with salt fish, onions and oil
Plantain	Can be sliced and fried (often eaten for Sunday breakfast). May be boiled and eaten as potatoes or put into soup
Green banana	Usually boiled
Yam	Available as white and yellow. May be boiled and eaten like potatoes or put into soup
Cassava	Has to be boiled (can be toxic if not); can be put into soup (eaten less often than yam)
Breadfruit	Similar to pumpkin, may be boiled or roasted
Pumpkin	Boiled and eaten with meal or put into soup
Cho cho or Christophene	Looks similar to hard green pear with a more flattened appearance. Can be boiled or put into soup
Sweet potato	Can be boiled or put into soup
Salt fish/salted cod	Bought dried, usually soaked overnight to remove salt or boiled to rehydrate before cooking
Salt fish fritters/fish cake	Salt fish pieces added into a batter and deep fried, may be home-made or bought from take-away
Ackee and salt fish	National dish of Jamaica. Ackee is oily fruit resembling scrambled eggs in appearance. Salt fish is fried and ackee added
White fish	Usually cooked with oil, onions and highly seasoned
Home-made West Indian soup	Made with meat, dumplings and large pieces of vegetables such as yam, sweet potato, pumpkin, carrots and cho cho in a thin stock. Usually eaten from a deep soup bowl
Curry lamb, beef, chicken, mutton and goat	Meat is usually seasoned overnight and then fried in oil. Water is added and the dish left to cook until tender. Creamed coconut may be added
Roast chicken, Oven do chicken	Meat is seasoned overnight. May be tossed in flour, then fried and cooked in oven
Pattie	Semi-circle of flavoured pastry filled with seasoned mince beef or vegetables. Eaten as snack usually from take-away
Rice and peas	Peas may be black-eyed peas, pigeon peas, kidney beans or split peas. Onions, vegetable oil and creamed coconut may be added
Fried dumplings or Johnny cake	Dough is made with white flour and deep fried. Home-made or take-away
Punch	Many different combinations; main ingredients listed below but subject to variation, e.g. Nutriment may be used to replace some of the condensed milk; spices used could include nutmeg, cinnamon, vanilla; fruit juice depending on personal preference Carrot juice punch: carrot juice, condensed milk, sugar and spices Fruit punch: fruit juice and fizzy pop Rum punch: rum and fruit juice Guinness punch: Guinness, condensed milk, egg, sugar and spices

Table 13. Foods defined as traditional West Indian foods

Hard dough bread	Cho Cho	Pattie
Sweet bun	Sweet potato	Rice and peas*
Cornmeal porridge	Saltfish fritters	Rice
Callaloo	Ackee and saltfish	Fried dumpling
Avocado pear	Home-made soup	Nutriment/Nourishment
Plantain	Oxtail stew	Curried chicken
Green banana	Fried chicken	Curried beef
Yam	Roast chicken (oven do)	Punch
Cassava	Roast pork (oven do)	Curried lamb/goat/mutton
Breadfruit	Roast lamb (oven do)	Pumpkin

*'Peas and rice' in Eastern Caribbean

Table 14. Percentage energy contributed by macronutrients for traditional and non-traditional eating – men and women

Nutrient as % of energy intake	Trad. males (*n* = 41)	Non-trad. males (*n* = 44)	Trad. females (*n* = 43)	Non-trad. females (*n* = 82)
Carbohydrate	53.9	51.0	53.0	51.9
CI	52.0–55.9	49.4–52.6	51.2–54.7	50.6–53.2
Of which alcohol	4.3	2.9	1.5	1.2
Fat	30.3	33.7	32.2	32.8
CI	28.5–32.0	32.4–35.0	30.7–33.7	31.7–34.0
Protein	15.1	14.7	14.4	14.8
CI	14.5–15.8	14.2–15.3	13.7–15.2	14.4–15.3

Source: Sharma, 1996

References

Abbotts, J, Williams, R, Ford, G, Hunt, K and West, P (1997). Morbidity and Irish Catholic descent in Britain: an ethnic and religious minority 150 years on. *Social Science and Medicine* **41**(1):3–14.

Abraham, R, Campbell-Brown, M, Haines, A P, North, W R S, Hainsworth, V and McFadyen, I R (1985). Diet during pregnancy in an Asian community in Britain – energy, protein, zinc, copper, fibre and calcium. *Human Nutrition: Applied Nutrition* **39A**:23–35.

Abraham, R, Campbell-Brown, M, North, W R S and McFadyen, I R (1987). Diets of Asian pregnant women in Harrow: iron and vitamins. *Human Nutrition: Applied Nutrition* **41A**:164–73.

Achaya, K T (1987). Fat status of Indians – a review. *Journal of Scientific and Industrial Research* **46**:112–26.

Agha, F, Sadaruddin, A, Khan, R A and Ghafoor, A (1992). Iron deficiency in adolescents. *Journal of the Pakistan Medical Association* **42**(1):3–5.

Ahmad, W I U (1989). Policies, pills and political will: a critique of policies to improve the health status of ethnic minorities. *Lancet* i:148–50.

Ahmad, W I U (1995). Review article: 'race' and health. *Sociology of Health & Sickness* **17**:418–29.

Ahmad, W I U, Kernohan, E E M and Baker, M R (1989). Health of British Asians: a research review. *Community Medicine* **11**(1):49–56.

Ahmad, W I U, Sheldon, T and Stuart, O (1996). Introduction. In Ahmad, W I U, Sheldon, T and Stuart, O (eds) *Ethnicity and health: reviews of literature and guidance for purchasers in the areas of cardiovascular disease, mental health and haemoglobinopathies*. CRD Report 5. York: NHS Centre for Reviews and Dissemination, pp. 25–104.

Ahmad, W I U and Walker, R (1997). Asian older people: housing, health and access to services. *Ageing and Society* **17**:141–65.

Ali, D and Begum, R A (1991). *Health and social circumstances of the elderly Bangladeshi population of Tower Hamlets: a background report*. London: Department of Health Care of the Elderly, Royal London Hospital Medical College, Royal London Hospital (Mile End).

Alleyne, S A, Cruickshank, J K, Golding, A L and Morrison, E Y St A (1989). Mortality from diabetes in Jamaica. *Bulletin of the Pan American Health Organization* **23**:306–15.

Allison, D B, Hoy, K, Fournier, A and Heymsfield, S B (1993). Can ethnic differences in men's preferences for women's body shapes contribute to ethnic differences in female obesity? *Obesity Research* **1**:425–32.

Allison, D B, Kanders, B S and Osage, G D (1995). Weight-related attitudes and beliefs of obese African American women. *Journal of Nutrition Education* **27**:18–23.

Anderson, A S and Lean, M E J (1995). Healthy changes? Observations on a decade of dietary change in a sample of Glaswegian South Asian migrant women. *Journal of Human Nutrition and Dietetics* **8**:129–36.

Anderson, A S, Lean, M E J, Bush, H, Bradby, H and Williams, R (1995). Macronutrient intake in South Asian and Italian women in the West of Scotland (abstract). *Proceedings of the Nutrition Society* **54**(3):203A.

Anon. (1976). *Asians in Britain: a study of their dietary patterns in relation to their cultural and religious backgrounds.* London: Van den Berghs and Jurgens.

—— (1986). *The Irish housewife: a portrait.* Dublin: Irish Consumer Research.

—— (1991). *Changing attitudes in Ireland.* Dublin: Behaviour and Attitudes Ltd, Institute of Advertising Practitioners in Ireland.

Armstrong, P L (1989). Iron deficiency in adolescents. *British Medical Journal* **298**:499.

Askham, J, Henshaw, L and Tarpey, M (1995). *Social and health authority services for elderly people from black and minority ethnic communities.* London: HMSO.

Aslam, M and Healy, M (1982). Present and future trends in the health care of British-Asian children. *Nursing Times,* 11 August:1353–54.

Aslam, M and Stockley, I H (1979). Interaction between curry ingredient (karela) and drug (chlorpropamide). *Lancet,* 17 March: vol. i 607.

Aspinall, P J (1996). *The development of an ethnic group question for the 2001 Census: the findings of a consultation exercise with members of the 2001 Census Working Subgroup on the Ethnic Group Question.* London: Office for National Statistics.

Atkin, K and Rollings, J (1993). *Community care in a multiracial Britain: a critical review of the literature.* London: HMSO.

Aukett, A and Wharton, B (1989). Nutrition of Asian children: infants and toddlers. In Cruickshank, J K and Beevers, D G (eds) *Ethnic factors in health and disease.* London: Wright, pp. 241–48.

Aykroyd, W R and Hussain, M A (1967). Diet and state of nutrition of Pakistani infants in Bradford, Yorkshire. *British Medical Journal* **1**:42–5.

Azuonye, I O (1996). Who is 'black' in medical research. *British Medical Journal* **313**:760.

Bahl, V (1987). *Asian Mother and Baby Campaign: director's report.* London: DHSS.

Bakhshi, S S (1993). Incidence of tuberculosis in England and Wales (rate in ethnic groups is decreasing). *British Medical Journal* **307**:865–6.

Balarajan, R (1995). Ethnicity and variations in the nation's health. *Health Trends* **27**:114–19.

Balarajan, R (1996). Ethnicity and variations in mortality from coronary heart disease. *Health Trends* **28**:45–51.

Balarajan, R and Bulusu, L (1990). Mortality among immigrants in England and Wales, 1979–83. In Britton, M (ed.) *Mortality and geography: a review in the mid-1980s.* London: HMSO.

Balarajan, R, Soni, R V and Botting, B (1989). Sudden infant death syndrome and postnatal mortality in immigrants in England and Wales. *British Medical Journal* **298**:716–20.

Ballard, R (1996). The Pakistanis: stability and introspection. In Peach, C (ed.) *Ethnicity in the 1991 Census,* vol. 2: The ethnic minority populations of Great Britain. London: HMSO, pp. 121–49.

Barker, M E, McClean, S I, McKenna, P G *et al.* (1989). *Diet, lifestyle and health in Northern Ireland.* Coleraine: Co. Londonderry Centre for Applied Health Studies, University of Ulster.

Barker, M E, McClean, S I, Thompson, K A and Reid, N G (1990). Dietary behaviours and sociocultural demographics in Northern Ireland. *British Journal of Nutrition* **64**:319–29.

Barker, M E, Thompson, K A and McClean, S I (1995). Attitudinal dimensions of food choice and nutrient intake. *British Journal of Nutrition* **74**:649–59.

Bashir, T, Macdonald, H N and Peacock, M (1981). Biochemical evidence of vitamin D deficiency in pregnant Asian women. *Journal of Human Nutrition* **35**:49–52.

Berrington, A (1994). Marriage and family formation among the white and ethnic minority populations in Britain. *Ethnic and Racial Studies* **17**(3):517–46.

Beshyah, S A, Jowett, N I and Burden, A C (1992). Metabolic control during Ramadan fasting. *Practical Diabetes* **9**(2):54–5.

Bhalla, A and Blakemore, K (1981). *Elders of the minority ethnic groups*. Birmingham: AFFOR.

Bhopal, R S (1986a). Asians' knowledge and behaviour on preventive health issues: smoking, alcohol, heart disease, pregnancy, rickets, malaria prophylaxis and surma. *Community Medicine* **8**(4):315–21.

—— (1986b). Bhye bhaddi: a food and health concept of Punjabi Asians. *Social Science and Medicine* **23**(7):687–8.

Bissenden, J G, Scott, P H, King, J, Hallum, J and Mansfield, H N (1981). Anthropometric and biochemical changes during pregnancy in Asian and European mothers having light for gestational age babies. *British Journal of Obstetrics and Gynaecology* **88**:999–1008.

Blakemore, K and Boneham, M (1994). *Age, race and ethnicity: a comparative approach*. Buckingham: Open University Press.

Bolton-Smith, C, Smith, W C S, Woodward, M, Brown, C A and Tunstall-Pedoe, H (1990). Dietary differences between social class groups in the Scottish Heart Health Study (abstract). *Proceedings of the Nutrition Society* **49**(1):62.

Boreham, C, Savage, J M, Primrose, D, Cran, G and Strain, J (1993). Coronary risk factors in schoolchildren. *Archives of Disease in Childhood* **68**:182–6.

Bose, K (1995). A comparative study of generalised obesity and anatomical distribution of subcutaneous fat in adult White and Pakistani migrant males in Peterborough. *Journal of the Royal Society of Health* **115**(2):90–5.

Box, V (1983). Rickets: what should the health education message be? *Health Visitor* **56**:131–4.

Bradby, H (1996). Cultural strategies of young women of South Asian origin in Glasgow, with special reference to health. Unpublished Ph.D. thesis, University of Glasgow.

Brah, A and Shaw, S (1992). *Working choices: South Asian young Muslim women and the labour market: a report for the Department of Employment*. Research Paper No. 91. London: Centre for Extra-Mural Studies, Birkbeck College.

Britton, M (1990). *Mortality and geography: a review in the mid-1980s*. London: HMSO.

Brooke, O G and Wood, C (1980). Growth in British Asians: longitudinal data in the first year. *Journal of Human Nutrition* **34**:355–9.

Brunvand, L, Henriksen, C, Larsson, M and Sandberg, A-S (1995). Iron deficiency among pregnant Pakistanis in Norway and the content of phytic acid in their diet. *Acta Obstetricia et Gynecologica Scandinavica* **74**:520–5.

Burke, G, Savage, P J, Manolio, T A, Sprafka, J M, Wagenknecht, L E, Sidney, S, Perkins, L L, Liu, K and Jacobs, D R (1992). Correlates of obesity in young Black and White women: the CARDIA study. *American Journal of Public Health* **82**:1621–5.

Burton-Jeangros, C (1995). Breast-feeding among mothers of Pakistani origin living in the UK. *Health Visitor* **68**(2):66–8.

Bush, H M and Williams, R G A (1995). Economic and cultural considerations in the food choice of South Asian and Italian women in the West of Scotland. Paper presented at Fourth Food Choice Conference, University of Birmingham, 24–26 April.

Bush, H M, Anderson, A S, Williams, R G A, Lean, M E J, Bradby, H and Abbotts, J (1995). *Dietary change in South Asian and Italian women in the West of Scotland.* MRC Medical Sociology Unit Working Paper No. 54. Glasgow: MRC Medical Sociology Unit.

Bush, H M, Williams, R G A, Bradby, H, Anderson, A and Lean, M E J (1998). Family hospitality and ethnic tradition among South Asian, Italian and general population women in the West of Scotland. *Sociology of Health and Illness* **20**(3):351–80.

Bush, H M, Williams, R G A, Bradby, H, Lean, M E J, Anderson, A S and Han, T (1996). Weight consciousness and body image among South Asian, Italian and general population women in Glasgow. Paper presented at the Society for Social Medicine 40th Annual Scientific Meeting, Dundee, 18–20 September.

Campbell-Brown, M, Ward, R J, Haines, A P, North, W R S, Abraham, R, McFadyen, I R, Turnlund, J R and King, J C (1985). Zinc and copper in Asian pregnancies – is there evidence for a nutritional deficiency? *British Journal of Obstetrics and Gynaecology* **92**:875–85.

Cappuccio, F and McGregor, G (1991). Meta-analysis of K+ supplements and blood pressure reduction trials. *Journal of Hypertension* **9**:465–74.

Carlson, E (1993). Adapting Foods. In Falshaw, M (ed.) *Beating heart disease: appropriate dietary advice for Afro-Caribbean, Bangladeshi and Chinese people.* Report of a one-day seminar: The Healthy Eastenders Project.

Caribbean Food and Nutrition Institute (1984). *Baseline survey of young child feeding practices.* Kingston, Jamaica: CFNI.

Carlson, E, Kipps, M and Thomson, J (1984). Influences on the food habits of some ethnic minorities in the United Kingdom. *Human Nutrition: Applied Nutrition* **38**:85–98.

Caulfield, B and Bhat, A (1981). The Irish in Britain: intermarriage and fertility levels 1971–1976. *New Community* **9**:73–83.

Chance, J (1996). The Irish: invisible settlers. In Peach, C (ed.) *Ethnicity in the 1991 Census,* vol. 2: The ethnic minority populations of Great Britain. London: HMSO, pp. 221–39.

Chandalia, H B and Bhargav, A (1987). Dietary pattern during Ramadan fasting and its effect on the metabolic control of diabetes. *Practical Diabetes* **4**:287–90.

Chaturvedi, N, McKeigue, P M and Marmot, M G (1993). Resting and ambulatory blood pressure in Afro-Caribbeans and Europeans. *Hypertension* **22**:90–6.

Chaturvedi, N and Fuller, J (1996). Ethnic differences in mortality from cardiovascular disease in the UK: do they persist in people with diabetes? *Journal of Epidemiology and Community Health* **50**:137–9.

Chaturvedi, N, Jarrett, J, Morrish, N, Keen, H and Fuller, J H (1996). Differences in mortality and morbidity in African-Caribbean and European people with non-insulin dependent diabetes mellitus: results of 20-year follow-up of a London cohort of a multinational study. *British Medical Journal* **313**:848–52.

Church, J and Summerfield, C (eds) (1996). *Social focus on ethnic majorities.* London: HMSO.

Clarson, C L, Barker, M J, Marshall, T and Wharton, B A (1982). Secular change in birthweight of Asian babies born in Birmingham. *Archives of Disease in Childhood* **57**:867–71.

Clements, M R (1989). The problem of rickets in UK Asians. *Journal of Human Nutrition and Dietetics* **2**:105–16.

Compton, P (1996). Indigenous and older minorities. In Coleman, D and Salt, J (eds) *Ethnicity in the 1991 Census,* vol. 1: Demographic characteristics of the ethnic minority populations. London: HMSO, pp. 243–82.

Conroy, R (1992). *The attitudes study.* Kilkenny Health Project in Newell, J, Nolan, G and Kelleher, C (1993).

Cooper, R S, Rotimi, C N, Kaufman, J S, Fraser, H, Forrester, T, Wolks, R, Riste, L K and Cruickshank, J K (1997). Prevalence of NIDDM among populations of the African diaspora. *Diabetes Care* **20**:343–8.

Cross, J H, Eminson, J and Wharton, B A (1990). Ramadan and birthweight at full term in Asian Moslem pregnant women in Birmingham. *Archives of Disease in Childhood* **65**:1053–6.

Cruickshank, J K (1989). Diabetes: contrasts between peoples of black (West African), Indian and white European origin. In Cruickshank, J K and Beevers, D G (eds) *Ethnic factors in health and disease*. London: Wright, pp. 289–304.

Cruickshank, J K (1993). The challenge of stroke and hypertension for the British Afro-Caribbean population. In *The health of the nation – the ethnic dimension*. London: Department of Health and NW/NE Thames RHA.

Cruickshank, J K (1995). Challenging the orthodoxy of insulin resistance. *Lancet* **346**:772–3.

Cruickshank, J K and Alleyne, S A (1987). Black West Indian and matched white diabetes in Britain compared with diabetics in Jamaica: blood pressure, body mass and vascular disease. *Diabetes Care* **10**:170–9.

Cruickshank, J K and Beevers, D G (1989). Migration, ethnicity, health and disease. In Cruickshank, J K and Beevers, D G (eds) *Ethnic factors in health and disease*. London: Wright, pp. 3–6.

Cruickshank, J K, Riste, L and Amica, C (1994). Rule of halves in hypertension control: how efforts in primary care can produce better results in Black than in White population samples. *Journal of Hypertension* **12**:1315.

Cruickshank, J K and Thompson, R L (unpublished). Nutrient intakes and typical foods eaten in a population sample of middle-aged Afro-Caribbean, White and Gujerati women living in West London.

Cruickshank, J K, Cooper, J, Burnett, M, MacDuff, J and Drubra, U (1991). Ethnic differences in fasting plasma C-peptide and insulin in relation to glucose tolerance and blood pressure. *Lancet* **333**:842–7.

Cruickshank, J K, Forrester, T, Mbanya, J C, Balkau, B, Riste, L, Jackson, M, Bennett, F and Wilks, R (1996). Standardized study of blood pressure in three African origin population samples in Cameroon, Jamaica and the UK. *Journal of Hypertension* **14** (suppl. 1) S236:1082.

Cruickshank, J K, Jackson, S H D, Beevers, D G, Bannan, L T, Beevers, M and Stewart, V L (1985). Similarity of blood pressure in Blacks, Whites and Asians in England: the Birmingham Factory Study. *Journal of Hypertension* **3**:365–71.

Currie, R, Gilbert, A and Horsley, L (1977). *Churches and churchgoers: patterns of church growth in the British Isles since 1700*. Oxford University Press.

Davies, D P, Senior, N, Cole, G, Blass, D and Simpson, K (1982). Size at birth of Asian and white Caucasian babies born in Leicester: implications for obstetric and paediatric practices. *Early Human Development* **6**:257–63.

Department of Health (1991). *Dietary reference values for food energy and nutrients for the United Kingdom: report of the Panel on Dietary Reference Values of the Committee on Medical Aspects of Food Policy*. Report on Health and Social Subjects 41. London: HMSO.

—— (1993). *Health of the Nation key area handbook: coronary heart disease and stroke*. London: Department of Health.

—— (1994a). *Nutritional aspects of cardiovascular disease: report of the Cardiovascular Review Group Committee on Medical Aspects of Food Policy*. Report on Health and Social Subjects 46. London: HMSO.

Department of Health (1994b). *Weaning and the weaning diet: report of the Working Group on the Weaning Diet of the Committee on Medical Aspects of Food Policy*. Report on Health and Social Subjects 45. London: HMSO.

Department of Health and Social Security (1980). *Rickets and osteomalacia*. Report on Health and Social Subjects 19. London: HMSO.

Dhawan, S (1995). Birth weights of infants of first generation Asian women in Britain compared with second generation Asian women. *British Medical Journal* **311**:86–8.

Di Giovanni, J V, Pentecost, B L, Beevers, D G, Beevers, M, Jackson, S H, Bannan, L T, Osbourne, V L and Mathews, K (1983). The Birmingham blood pressure school study. *Postgraduate Medical Journal* **59**(696):627–9.

Dineen, B (1992). Consumer food choice, socioeconomic profile and retail provision in two Galway supermarkets serving different socioeconomic areas. Paper presented at the Nutrition Society Irish Group Postgraduate Seminar Series, Galway.

Dobson, S M (1988). Transcultural health visiting: caring in a multi-cultural society. *Recent Advances in Nursing* **20**:61–80.

Donaldson, L J (1986). Health and social status of elderly Asians: a community survey. *British Medical Journal* **293**:1079–82.

Donnison, J (1993). Developing strategies for change: issues involved in enabling people to change their diets in order to reduce serum cholesterol. In Falshaw, M (ed.) *Beating heart disease: appropriate dietary advice for Afro-Caribbean, Bangladeshi and Chinese people*. Report of a one-day seminar. The Healthy Eastenders Project.

Donovan, J L (1984). Ethnicity and health: a research review. *Social Science and Medicine* **19**(7):663–70.

Douglas, J (1987). *Caribbean food and diet*. Cambridge: National Extension College for Training in Health and Race.

Douglas, J (1989). Food type preferences and trends among Afro-Caribbeans in Britain. In Cruickshank, J K and Beevers, D G (eds) *Ethnic factors in health and disease*. London: Wright, pp. 249–54.

Douglas, J (1993). Developing a multiracial perspective in preventing heart disease. In Falshaw, M (ed.) *Beating heart disease: appropriate dietary advice for Afro-Caribbean, Bangladeshi and Chinese people*. Report of a one-day seminar. The Healthy Eastenders Project.

Dowler, E and Calvert, C (1995). *Nutrition and diet in lone parent families in London*. London: Family Policy Studies Centre.

Draper, E S, Abrams, K R and Clarke, M (1995). Fall in birth weight of third generation Asian infants (letter). *British Medical Journal* **311**:876.

Duggan, M B, Steel, G, Elwys, G, Harbottle, L and Noble, C (1991). Iron status, energy intake, and nutritional status of healthy young Asian children. *Archives of Disease in Childhood* **66**:1386–9.

Dunnigan, M G, Glekin, B M, Henderson, J B, McIntosh, W B, Sumner, D and Sutherland, G R (1985). Prevention of rickets in Asian children: assessment of the Glasgow campaign. *British Medical Journal* **291**:239–42.

Dunnigan, M G, Paton, J P J, Haase, S, McNicol, G W, Gardner, M D and Smith, C M (1962). Late rickets and osteomalacia in the Pakistani community in Glasgow. *Scottish Medical Journal*, **7**:159–67.

Eade, J (1989). East End Muslims. *The Tablet*, 18 March.

Eade, J, Vamplew, T and Peach, C (1996). The Bangladeshis: the encapsulated community. In Peach, C (ed.) *Ethnicity in the 1991 Census*, vol. 2: The ethnic minority populations of Great Britain. London: HMSO, pp. 150–60.

Eaton, P M, Wharton, P A and Wharton, B A (1984). Nutrient intake of pregnant Asian women at Sorrento Maternity Hospital, Birmingham. *British Journal of Nutrition* **52**:457–68.

Ebrahim, S, Patel, N, Coats, M, Greig, C, Gilley, J, Bangham, C and Stacey, S (1991). Prevalence and severity of morbidity among Gujarati Asian elders: a controlled comparison. *Family Practice* **8**(1):57–62.

Ehrhardt, P (1986). Iron deficiency in young Bradford children from different ethnic groups. *British Medical Journal* **292**:90–3.

Evans, A E, Ruidavets, J-B, McCrum, E E, Cambou, J-P, McClean, R, Douste-Blazy, P, McMaster, D, Bingham, A, Patterson, C C, Richard, J L, Mathewson, Z M and Cambien, F (1995). Autres pays, autres coeurs? Dietary patterns, risk factors and ischaemic heart disease in Belfast and Toulouse. *Quarterly Journal of Medicine* **88**:469–77.

Falshaw, M (ed.) (1993). *Beating heart disease: appropriate dietary advice for Afro-Caribbean, Bangladeshi and Chinese people*. Report of a one-day seminar. The Healthy Eastenders Project.

Finch, P J, Ang, L, Eastwood, J B and Maxwell, J D (1992). Clinical and histological spectrum of osteomalacia among Asians in South London. *Quarterly Journal of Medicine* **83**(302):439–48.

Finch, P J, Millard, F J C and Maxwell, J D (1991). Risk of tuberculosis in immigrant Asians: culturally acquired immunodeficiency? *Thorax* **46**:1–5.

Flood, P (1993). A healthy diet for adults. *World of Irish Nursing* **1**(1):32–3.

Ford, J A (1974). Asian rickets and osteomalacia. *Nursing Times* **70**(2):49–50.

Ford, J A, Colhoun, E M, McIntosh, W B and Dunnigan, M G (1972). Rickets and osteomalacia in the Glasgow Pakistani Community, 1961–71. *British Medical Journal* **2**:677–80.

Forrest, R D, Jackson, C A and Yudkin, J S (1986). Glucose intolerance and hypertension in North London: the Islington Survey. *Diabetic Medicine* **3**:338–42.

Fowler, H, Griffin, E, Lawton, F, Buxton, J and Luesley, D (1990). Antenatal attendance and fasting of pregnant Muslims during Ramadan. *British Journal of Obstetrics and Gynaecology* **97**:861–2.

Frayn, K N, Williams, C M and Arner, P (1996). Are increased non-esterified fatty acid concentrations a risk marker for coronary heart disease and other chronic diseases? *Clinical Science* **90**:243–53.

Friel, S, Nolan, G and Kelleher, C (1995). *Health status of the Irish population 1994*. Galway: National Nutrition Surveillance Centre, Centre for Health Promotion Studies, University College, Galway.

Ganatra, S (1989). Features of Gujarati, Punjabi and Muslim diets in the UK. In Cruickshank, J K and Beevers, D G (eds) *Ethnic factors in health and disease*. London: Wright, pp. 227–30.

Garrow, J S (1982). *Treating obesity seriously: a clinical manual*. London: Churchill.

Gibney, M J and Lee, P (1989). *Patterns of food and nutrient intake in a suburb of Dublin with chronically high unemployment*. Combat Poverty Agency Report Series No. 2.

Gibney, M J, Moloney, M and Shelley, E (1989). The Kilkenny Health Project: food and nutrient intakes in randomly selected healthy adults. *British Journal of Nutrition* **61**:129–37.

Gishen, F S, Hogh, L M and Stock, M J (1995). Differences in conicity in young adults of European and South Asian descent. *International Journal of Obesity* **19**:146–8.

Goel, K M (1979). *Nutrition survey of immigrant children in Glasgow.* Scottish Health Service Studies, No. 40. Edinburgh: HMSO.

Goodwin, A M, Keen, H and Mather, H M (1987). Ethnic minorities in British diabetic clinics: a questionnaire survey. *Diabetic Medicine* **4**:266–9.

Great Britain Working Party on Fortification of Food with Vitamin D (1980). *Rickets and osteomalacia: report of the Working Party on Fortification of Food with Vitamin D.* Committee on Medical Aspects of Food Policy. London: HMSO.

Gregory, J, Foster, K, Tyler, H and Wiseman, M (1990). *The dietary and nutritional survey of British adults.* London: HMSO.

Griffiths, K (1983). Child-rearing practices in West Indian, Indian and Pakistani communities. *New Community* **10**(3):393–409.

Grindulis, H, Scott, P H, Belton, N R and Wharton, B A (1986). Combined deficiency of iron and vitamin D in Asian toddlers. *Archives of Disease in Childhood* **61**:843–8.

Habba, S F and Doyle, J S (1982). Large bowel cancer: an Irish epidemic? *Irish Medical Journal* **75**(11):439–40.

Habba, S F, Daly, L and Doyle, J S (1982). Epidemiology of carcinoma of the colon and rectum in Ireland: mortality analysis. *Irish Journal of Medical Science* **151**:6–11.

Harbottle, L and Duggan, M B (1992). Comparative study of the dietary characteristics of Asian toddlers with iron deficiency in Sheffield. *Journal of Human Nutrition and Dietetics* **5**:351–61.

Harding, S and Balarajan, R (1996). Patterns of mortality in second generation Irish living in England and Wales: longitudinal study. *British Medical Journal* **312**:1389–92.

Harris, R J, Armstrong, D, Ali, R and Loynes A (1983). Nutritional survey of Bangladeshi children aged under 5 years in the London borough of Tower Hamlets. *Archives of Disease in Childhood* **58**:428–32.

Hawthorne, K, Mello, M and Tomlinson, S (1993). Cultural and religious influences in diabetes care in Great Britain. *Diabetic Medicine* **10**:8–12.

Henderson, J B, Dunnigan, M G, McIntosh, W B, Motaal, A A and Hole, D (1990). Asian osteomalacia is determined by dietary factors when exposure to ultraviolet radiation is restricted: a risk factor model. *Quarterly Journal of Medicine* **76**(281):923–33.

Henderson, J B, Glekin, B M, McIntosh, W B and Dunnigan, M G (1989). A health education campaign to prevent osteomalacia in Asian women in Glasgow: 1984–86. *Journal of Human Nutrition and Dietetics* **2**:237–51.

Henriksen, C, Brunvand, L, Stoltenberg, C, Trygg, K, Haug, E and Pedersen, J I (1995). Diet and vitamin D status among pregnant Pakistani women in Oslo. *European Journal of Clinical Nutrition* **49**:211–18.

Henson, S (1992). From high street to hypermarket. In National Consumer Council (ed.) *Your food: Whose choice?* London: HMSO, pp. 95–115.

Hickman, M. (1995). *Religion, class and identity: the state, the Catholic Church and the education of the Irish in Britain.* Aldershot: Avebury.

Hilder, A S(1994). Ethnic differences in the sudden infant death syndrome: what we can learn from immigrants to the UK. *Early Human Development* **38**:143–9.

Hill, S E (ed.) (1987). *Report of the Food and Black and Ethnic Minorities Conference.* London: The London Food Commission.

Homans, H (1983). A question of balance: Asian and British women's perceptions of food during pregnancy. In Murcott, A (ed.) *The sociology of food and eating*. Aldershot: Gower, pp. 73–83.

Hope, A and Kelleher, C (1995). *Health at Work*. Centre for Health Promotion Studies. University College Galway: Galway, Ireland.

Hornsby-Smith, M and Dale, A (1988). The assimilation of Irish immigrants in England. *British Journal of Sociology* **39**:519–43.

Iqbal, S J, Kaddam, I, Wassif, W, Nichol, F and Walls, J (1994). Continuing clinically severe vitamin D deficiency in Asians in the UK (Leicester). *Postgraduate Medical Journal* **70**:708–14.

Irish Nutrition and Dietetic Institute (1990). *The Irish National Nutrition Survey*. Dublin: Irish Nutrition and Dietetic Institute.

James, J and Laing, G (1994). Iron deficiency anaemia. *Current Paediatrics* **4**:33–7.

Jones, T (1993). *Britain's ethnic minorities: an analysis of the Labour Force Survey*. London: Policy Studies Institute.

Jones, V M (1987). Current infant weaning practices within the Bangladeshi community in the London borough of Tower Hamlets. *Human Nutrition: Applied Nutrition* **41A**:349–52.

Kalka, I (1988). The changing food habits of Gujaratis in Britain. *Journal of Human Nutrition and Dietetics* **1**:329–35.

Kanders, B, Ullman-Joy, P, Foreyt, J P, Heymsfield, S B, Herber, D, Elashoff, R M, Ashley, J M, Reeves, R S and Blackburn, G L (1994). The Black American Lifestyle Intervention (BALI): the design of a weight loss program for working-class African-American women. *Journal of the American Dietetic Association* **3**:310–12.

Karmi, G and McKeigue, P M (1993). *The ethnic health bibliography*. London: NE and NW Thames RHA.

Kassam-Khamis, T, Judd, P, Thomas, J E, Sevak, L, Reddy, S and Ganatra, S (1995). Frequency of consumption and nutrient composition of composite dishes commonly consumed by South Asians originating from Gujerat and the Punjab. *Journal of Human Nutrition and Dietetics* **8**:265–77.

Kassam-Khamis, T, Thomas, J E and Judd, P (1996). Eating habits of second generation South Asians in the UK. *Scandinavian Journal of Nutrition* **40**:S84–S86.

Kearney, M and Gibney, M J (1993). Dietary beliefs and practices of a cross-section of the adult population and a supplement-using subgroup (abstract). Paper presented at Irish Nutrition and Dietetic Institute Annual Study Day.

Kemm, J, Douglas, J and Sylvester, V (1986). A survey of infant feeding practices by African-Caribbean Mothers in Birmingham. *Proceedings of the Nutrition Society* **45**:87a.

Kelleher, D and Islam, S (1994). The problem of integration: Asian people and diabetes. *Journal of the Royal Society of Medicine* **87**:414–17.

Khajuria, S and Thomas, J (1992). Traditional Indian beliefs about the dietary management of diabetes – an exploratory study of the implications for the management of Gujarati diabetics in Britain. *Human Nutrition and Dietetics* **5**:311–21.

Khaw, K T and Marmot, M G (1983). Blood pressure in 15 to 16 year old adolescents of different ethnic groups in two London schools. *Postgraduate Medical Journal* **59**:630–1.

King, H and Dowd, J E (1990). Primary prevention of type 2 (non-insulin-dependent) diabetes mellitus. *Diabetologia* **33**:3–8.

Knight, T M, Smith, Z, Whittles, A, Sahota, P, Lockton, J A, Hogg, G, Bedford, A, Toop, M, Kernohan, E E M and Baker, M R (1992). Insulin resistance, diabetes, and risk markers for ischaemic heart disease in Asian men and non-Asian men in Bradford. *British Heart Journal* **67**:343–50.

Korlipara, K (1995). Dealing with diabetes in Asians. *Geriatric Medicine* **25**:12.

Kumanyika, S K (1995). Nutrition and health campaign for all women. *Journal of the American Dietetic Association* **95**:299–300.

Kumanyika, S K, Obarzanek, E, Stevens, V J, Hebert, P R and Whelton, P K (1991). Weight loss experience of black and white participants in NHLBI sponsored clinical trials. *American Journal of Clinical Nutrition* **53**:1631S–1638S.

Kumanyika, S K, Wilson, J and Guilford-Davenport, M (1993). Weight-related attitudes and behaviors of black women. *Journal of the American Dietetic Association* **93**:416–22.

Kushi, L H, Lew, R A, Stare, F J et al. (1985). Diet and 20-year mortality from coronary heart disease: the Ireland–Boston Diet–Heart Study. *New England Journal of Medicine* **312**(13):811–17.

Landman, J and Wyke, S (1995). *Healthy eating and South Asian families in Scotland.* Edinburgh: Health Education Board for Scotland.

Lane, A, Cruickshank, J K, Mitchell, J, Henderson, A, Humphries, S and Green, F (1992). Genetic and environmental determinants of factor VII coagulant activity in ethnic groups at differing risk of coronary heart disease. *Atherosclerosis* **94**:43–50.

Lip, G Y H, Malik, I, Luscombe, C, McCarry, M and Beevers, G (1995). Dietary fat purchasing habits in whites, blacks and Asian peoples in England – implications for heart disease prevention. *International Journal of Cardiology* **48**:287–93.

Low Income Project Team for the Nutrition Task Force (1996). *Low income, food, nutrition and health: strategies for improvement.* London: Department of Health.

Lowry, M and Lillis, D F (1993). Infant feeding practices. *Irish Medical Journal* **86**(1):13–14.

Mangtani, P, Jolley, D J, Watson, J M and Rodrigues, L C (1995). Socioeconomic deprivation and notification rates for tuberculosis in London during 1982–91. *British Medical Journal* **310**:963–6.

Manolio, T A, Burke, G L, Psaty, B M, Newman, A B, Haan, M, Powe, N, Tracey, R P and O'Leary, D H (1995). Black–white differences in subclinical cardiovascular disease among older adults: the Cardiovascular Health Study. *Journal of Clinical Epidemiology* **48**:1141–52.

Marmot, M G, Adelstein, A ·M and Bulusu, L (1984). *Immigrant mortality in England and Wales.* London: HMSO.

Martorell, R (1985). Child growth retardation: a discussion of its causes and its relationship to health. In Blaxter, K and Waterlow, J C (eds) *Nutritional adaptation in man.* London: John Libbey, pp. 13–30.

Mason, E S, Davies, D P and Marshall, W A (1982). Early postnatal weight gain: comparisons between Asian and white Caucasian infants. *Early Human Development* **6**:253–5.

Mayor, V (1984). Pregnancy, childbirth and child care. *Nursing Times* **80**(24):57–8.

Mays, N (1983). Elderly South Asians in Britain: a survey of relevant literature and themes for future research. *Ageing and Society* **3**(1):71–97.

Mbanya, J C, Wilks, R, Bennett, F, Jackson, M, Forrester, T, Riste, L, Forhan, A, Balkau, B and Cruickshank, J K (in press). Standardised study of glucose tolerance and diabetes prevalence in four African (origin) populations in Cameroon, Jamaica and migrants to Britain. *Diabetologia*.

McCluskey D (1989). *Health – people's beliefs and practices*. Dublin: Government Stationery Office.

McEnery, G and Rao, K P S (1986). The effectiveness of antenatal education of Pakistani and Indian women living in this country. *Child: Care, Health and Development* **12**:385–99.

McFadyen, I R, Campbell-Brown, M, Abraham, R, North, W R S and Haines, A P (1984). Factors affecting birthweights in Hindus, Moslems and Europeans. *British Journal of Obstetrics and Gynaecology* **91**:968–72.

McGinn, T (1989). The baby and the bath-water. *Health Visitor* **62**:125.

McKeigue, P M and Chaturvedi, N (1996). Epidemiology and control of cardiovascular disease in South Asians and Afro-Caribbeans. In Ahmad, W, Sheldon, T and Stuart, O (eds) *Ethnicity and health: reviews of literature and guidance for purchasers in the areas of cardiovascular disease, mental health and haemoglobinopathies*. CRD Report 5. York: NHS Centre for Reviews and Dissemination, pp. 25–104.

McKeigue, P M, Marmot, M G, Adelstein, A M, Hunt, S P, Shipley, M J, Butler, S M, Riemersma, R A and Turner, P R (1985). Diet and risk factors for coronary heart disease in Asians in north-west London. *Lancet* ii:1086–90.

McKeigue, P M, Marmot, M G, Syndercombe Court, Y D, Courier, D E, Rahman, S and Riemersma, R A (1988). Diabetes, hyperinsulinaemia and coronary risk factors in Bangladeshis in east London. *British Heart Journal* **60**:390–6.

McKeigue, P M, Miller, G J and Marmot, M G (1989). Coronary heart disease in South Asians overseas: a review. *Journal of Clinical Epidemiology* **42**:597–609.

McKeigue, P M and Sevak, L (1994). *Coronary heart disease in South Asian communities: a manual for health promotion*. London: Health Education Authority.

McKeigue, P M, Shah, B and Marmot, M G (1991). Relation of central obesity and insulin resistance with high diabetes prevalence and cardiovascular risk in South Asians. *Lancet* **337**:382–6.

McNabb, W L, Quinn, M T and Rosing, L (1993). Weight loss program for inner-city black women with non-insulin-dependent diabetes mellitus. *Journal of the American Dietetic Association* **93**:75–7.

McNeill, G (1985). Birth weight, feeding practices and weight-for-age of Punjabi children in the UK and in the rural Punjab. *Human Nutrition: Clinical Nutrition* **39C**:69–72.

McSweeney, M and Kevany, J (1982). A national survey of infant feeding practices in Ireland 1981: a preliminary report. *Irish Medical Journal* **75**(12):452–5.

Meade, T W, Brozovic, M and Chakaborti, R (1978). Ethnic group comparisons of variable associated with ischaemic heart disease. *British Heart Journal* **40**:789–95.

Meikle, J (1996). Asian corner shop faces extinction. *The Guardian*, 17 September.

Melynk, M and Weinstein, E (1994). Preventing obesity in black women by targetting adolescents: a literature review. *Journal of the American Dietetic Association* **94**:536–40.

Miller, G J, Kotecha, S, Wilkinson, W H, Wilkes, H, Stirling, Y, Sanders, T A B, Broadhurst, A, Allison, J and Meade, T,W (1988). Dietary and other characteristics relevant for coronary heart disease in men of Indian, West Indian and European descent in London. *Atherosclerosis* **70**:63–72.

Moore, A and Worwood, M (1989). Iron and the sudden infant death syndrome. *British Medical Journal* **298**:1248.

Morgan, M (1995). The significance of ethnicity for health promotion: patients' use of anti-hypertensive drugs in inner London. *International Journal of Epidemiology* **24** (suppl. 1):S79–S84.

Morrison, E and Richards, R (1985). Clinical profile of diabetes mellitus in Jamaica (phasic insulin dependence). *West Indian Medical Journal* **34**:94–7.

Mulliner, C M, Spiby, H and Fraser, R B (1995). A study exploring midwives' education in, knowledge of and attitudes to nutrition in pregnancy. *Midwifery* **11**:37–41.

Murphy, M (1996). Household and family structure among ethnic minority groups. In Coleman, D and Salt, J (eds) *Ethnicity in the 1991 Census*, vol. 1: Demographic characteristics of the ethnic minority populations. London: HMSO, pp. 213–41.

Nelson, M, Bakaliou, F and Trivedi, A (1994). Iron-deficiency anaemia and physical performance in adolescent girls from different ethnic backgrounds. *British Journal of Nutrition* **72**:427–33.

Newell, J, Nolan, G and Kelleher, C (1993). *Nutritional surveillance in Ireland 1993*. Galway: Galway Centre for Health Promotion Studies, University College, Galway.

Nutrition Standing Committee of the British Paediatric Association (1988). Vegetarian weaning. *Archives of Disease in Childhood* **63**:1286–92.

Odugbesan, O, Rowe, B, Fletcher, J, Walford, S and Barnett, A H (1989). Diabetes in the UK West Indian community in Wolverhampton. *British Medical Journal* **6**:48–52.

Office of Population Censuses and Surveys/General Register for Scotland (1994). *1991 Census: ethnic group and country of birth: Great Britain*. London: HMSO.

O'Reilly, O and Shelley, E (1991). The Kilkenny post-primary schools survey – a survey of knowledge, attitudes and behaviour relevant to non-communicable diseases. *Irish Journal of Medical Science* **160** (suppl. 9): 40–4.

Ormerod, L P, Nunn, A J, Byfield, S P and Darbyshire, J H (1991). Patterns of tuberculosis in Indian and Pakistani/Bangladeshi patients: effects of age, date of first entry and ethnic group. *Respiratory Medicine* **85**:275–80.

Owen, D (1994a). *South Asian people in Great Britain: social and economic circumstances. 1991 Census Statistical Paper No. 7*. Warwick: Centre for Research in Ethnic Relations, University of Warwick.

Owen, D (1994b). *Black people in Great Britain: social and economic circumstances. 1991 Census Statistical Paper No. 6*. Warwick: Centre for Research in Ethnic Relations, University of Warwick.

Owen, D (1995). *Irish-born people in Great Britain: social and economic circumstances. 1991 Census Statistical Paper No. 9*. Warwick: Centre for Research in Ethnic Relations, University of Warwick.

Owen, D (1996). *Towards 2001: ethnic minorities and the Census*. Warwick: Centre for Research in Ethnic Relations, University of Warwick.

Passmore, R and Eastwood, M A (1986). *Davidson and Passmore Human Nutrition and Dietetics*. 8th edn. Edinburgh: Churchill Livingstone.

Peach, H (1984). A review of aetiological and intervention studies on rickets and osteomalacia in the United Kingdom. *Community Medicine* **6**:119–26.

Peach, C (1996). Introduction. In Peach, C (ed.) *Ethnicity in the 1991 Census*, vol. 2: The ethnic minority populations of Great Britain. London: HMSO, pp. 1–24.

Pearson, M, Madden, M and Greenslade, L (1991). *Generations of an invisible minority*. University of Liverpool, Institute of Irish Studies.

Peterson, D B, Dattani, J, Baylis, J M and Jepson, E M (1986). Dietary practices of Asian diabetics. *British Medical Journal* **292**:170–1.

Potrykus, C (1991). Time for action on black health. *Health Visitor* **64**:283–5.

Potts, J and Simmons, D (1994). Sex and ethnic group differences in fat distribution in young UK South Asians and Europids. *Journal of Clinical Epidemiology* **47**(8):837–41.

Proudler, A J, Godsland, I F, Bruce, M, Seed, M and Wynn, V (1996). Lipid and carbohydrate metabolic risk markers for coronary heart disease and blood pressure in healthy non-obese premenopausal women of different racial origins in the United Kingdom. *Metabolism* **45**(3):328–33.

Raftery, J, Jones, D R and Rosato, M (1990). The mortality of first and second generation Irish immigrants in the UK. *Social Science and Medicine* **31**(5):577–84.

Raman, A V (1988). Traditional practices and nutritional taboos. *Nursing Journal of India* LXXIX(6):143–5.

Rashed, A H (1992). The fast of Ramadan. *British Medical Journal* **304**:521–2.

Reddy, S and Sanders, T A B (1992). Lipoprotein risk factors in vegetarian women of Indian descent are unrelated to dietary intake. *Atherosclerosis* **95**:223–9.

Riddoch, C, Savage, J M, Murphy, N, Cran, G W and Boreham, C (1991). Long-term health implications of fitness and physical activity patterns. *Archives of Disease in Childhood* **66**:1426–33.

Riste, L K (1997). Risk factors associated with glucose tolerance and high blood pressure among African-Caribbean and white populations in Manchester: opportunities for prevention. Unpublished Ph.D. thesis, University of Manchester.

Robertson, I, Glekin, B M, Henderson, J B, McIntosh, W B, Lakhani, A and Dunnigan, M G, (1982). Nutritional deficiencies among ethnic minorities in the United Kingdom. *Proceedings of the Nutrition Society* **41**:243–55.

Robertson, J A and Kevany, J J (1982). Trends in the availability of foods for human consumption in Ireland. *Irish Journal of Medical Science* **151**(9):272–8.

Robinson, V (1996). The Indians: onward and upward. In Peach, C (ed.) *Ethnicity in the 1991 Census*, vol. 2: The ethnic minority populations of Great Britain. London: HMSO, pp. 95–119.

Rocheron, Y (1988). The Asian Mother and Baby Campaign: the construction of ethnic minorities' health needs. *Critical Social Policy*, **8**:4–23.

Rocheron, Y and Dickinson, R (1990). The Asian Mother and Baby Campaign: a way forward in health promotion for Asian women? *Health Education Journal* **49**(3);128–33.

Rocheron, Y, Dickinson, R and Khan, S (1988). *The evaluation of the Asian Mother and Baby Campaign: 1. Assessment of the Linkwork scheme*. Leicester: Centre for Mass Communication Research, University of Leicester.

Rocheron, Y, Dickinson, R and Khan, S (1989a). *The evaluation of the Asian Mother and Baby Campaign: 2. The before and after survey*. Leicester: Centre for Mass Communication Research, University of Leicester.

Rocheron, Y, Dickinson, R and Khan, S (1989b). *The evaluation of the Asian Mother and Baby Campaign: full summary*. Leicester: Centre for Mass Communication Research, University of Leicester.

Rocheron, Y, Dickinson, R and Khan, S (1989c). *The evaluation of the Asian Mother and Baby Campaign: synopsis*. Leicester: Centre for Mass Communication Research, University of Leicester.

Rona, R J, Chinn, S, Duggal, S and Driver, A P (1987). Vegetarianism and growth in Urdu, Gujarati and Punjabi children in Britain. *Journal of Epidemiology and Community Health* **41**:233–6.

Royal College of Physicians of London (1983). Obesity. *Journal of the Royal College of Physicians* **17**:5–65.

Rudat, K (1994). *Black and minority ethnic groups in England: health and lifestyles*. London: Health Education Authority.

Sahota, P (1991). *Feeding baby: inner city practice*. Bradford: Horton Publishing.

Samanta, A, Campbell, J E, Spaulding, D L, Neogi, S K, Panja, K K and Burden, A C (1986). Eating habits in Asian diabetics. *Diabetic Medicine* **3**(3):283–4.

Save the Children Fund (1983). *Stop Rickets Campaign – report of a health education campaign*. London: DHSS.

Sevak, L, McKeigue, P M and Marmot, M G (1994). Relation of hyperinsulinemia to dietary intake in South Asian and European men. *American Journal of Clinical Nutrition* **59**:1069–74.

Shahjahan, M (1991). Infant and toddler feeding patterns and related issues in the Bangladeshi community. Unpublished M.Sc. thesis, Department of Child Health, University of Newcastle.

Sharma, A (1990). Hypoglycaemic effects of fenugreek seeds in non-insulin dependent subjects. *Nutrition Research* **10**(7):731–9.

Sharma, S (1996). Developing food frequency questionnaires to assess nutrient intakes in African-origin populations in Cameroon, Jamaica and the UK. Unpublished Ph.D. thesis, University of Manchester.

Sharma, S, Cade, J E and Cruickshank, J K (1993). An initial assessment of food and nutrient intake for the development of a food frequency questionnaire for use in an Afro-Caribbean population sample. *Proceedings of the Nutrition Society* **52**(3):328A.

Sharma, S, Cade, J, Griffiths, S and Cruickshank, J K (1998). Nutrient intakes among UK African-Caribbean people: changing risk of coronary heart disease? *Lancet* **352**:114–15.

Sharma, S, Jackson, M, Mbanya, J C, Cade, J E, Forrester, T, Wilks, R, Balkau, B and Cruickshank, J K (1996). Development of food frequency questionnaires in three population samples of African origin from Cameroon, Jamaica and Caribbean migrants to the UK. *European Journal of Clinical Nutrition* **50**:479–86.

Shaukat, N, de Bono, D P and Jones, D R (1994). Like father like son? Sons of patients of European or Indian origin with coronary artery disease reflect their parents' risk factor pattern. *British Heart Journal* **74**:318–23.

Shaunak, S, Colston, K, Ang, L, Patel, S P and Maxwell, J D (1985). Vitamin D deficiency in adult British Hindu Asians: a family disorder. *British Medical Journal* **291**:1166–8.

Sheikh, N and Thomas, J (1994a). Factors influencing food choice among ethnic minority adolescents. *Nutrition and Food Science* **4**:18–22.

—— (1994b). Factors influencing food choice among ethnic minority adolescents. *Nutrition and Food Science* **5**:29–35.

Shelley, E, Daly, L, Collins, C *et al.* (1995). Cardiovascular risk factor changes in the Kilkenny Health Project. *European Heart Journal* **16**:752–60.

Shelley, E, Daly, L, Graham I *et al.* (1991a). The Kilkenny Health Project: a community research and demonstration cardiovascular health programme. *Irish Journal of Medical Science* 160 (suppl. 9):10–16.

Shelley, E, Daly, L, Kilcoyne, D and Graham, I (1991b). Obesity: a public health problem in Ireland? *Irish Journal of Medical Science* 160 (suppl. 9):29–34.

Sher, K S, Fraser, R C, Wicks, A C and Mayberry, J F (1993). High risk of coeliac disease in Punjabis. *Digestion* **54**:178–82.

Shukla, K (1987). Which diet is healthy? In Hill, S E (ed.) *Report of the Food and Black and Ethnic Minorities Conference*. London: London Food Commission.

Shukla, K (1991). Nutrition and dietetics. In Squires, A (ed.) *Multicultural health care and rehabilitation of older people*. London: Edward Arnold.

Silman, A, Loysen, E, de Graaf, W and Sramek, M (1985). High dietary fat intake and cigarette smoking as risk factors for ischaemic heart disease in Bangladeshi male immigrants in East London. *Journal of Epidemiology and Community Health* **39**:301–3.

Singleton, N and Tucker, S M (1978). Vitamin D status of Asian infants. *British Medical Journal* **1**:607–10.

Smith, R (1990). Asian rickets and osteomalacia. *Quarterly Journal of Medicine* **76**(281):899–901.

Smith, Z, Knight, T, Sahota, P, Kernohan, E and Baker, M (1993). Dietary patterns in Asian and Caucasian men in Bradford: differences and implications for nutrition education. *Journal of Human Nutrition and Dietetics* **6**:323–33.

Smithells, D (1996). Vitamins in early pregnancy. *British Medical Journal* **313**:128–19.

Sobal, J and Stunkard, A J (1989). Socioeconomic status and obesity: a review of the literature. *Psychological Bulletin* **105**(2):260–75.

Solanki, T, Hyatt, R H, Kemm, J R, Hughes, E A and Cowan, R A (1995). Are elderly Asians in Britain at a high risk of vitamin D deficiency and osteomalacia? *Age and Ageing* **24**:103–7.

South, J (1993). Meeting the needs of Asian patients. *Practice Nursing* **4**:10.

Squires, A (ed.) (1991). *Multicultural health care and rehabilitation of older people*. London: Edward Arnold.

Stephens, W P, Klimiuk, P S and Warrington, S (1981). Preventing vitamin D deficiency in immigrants: is encouragement enough? (letter) *Lancet* 25 April: 945–6.

Stephens, W P, Klimiuk, P S, Warrington, S and Taylor, J L (1982). Observations on the dietary practices of Asians in the United Kingdom. *Human Nutrition: Applied Nutrition* **36A**:438–44.

Strachan, D P, Powell, K J, Thaker, A, Millard, F J C and Maxwell, J D (1995). Vegetarian diet as a risk factor for tuberculosis in immigrant south London Asians. *Thorax* **50**:175–80.

Tauber, I J, Ali, R, Bishop, M, Forest, D, Halpern, P, Kapadia, M, Leonore, C S F and Loynes, A (1980). Preliminary results of a picture recognition study amongst Bangladeshi women. *Health Visitor* **53**:251–3.

Thalayasing, B (1985). Coeliac disease as a cause of osteomalacia and rickets in the Asian immigrant population. *British Medical Journal* **290**:1146–7.

Thomas, M and Avery, V (1997). *Infant feeding in Asian families*. Office for National Statistics. London: HMSO.

Thompson, R and Cruickshank, J K (1990). Dietary fatty acid intakes and P:S ratios in a population sample of women with different coronary risks (abstract). *Clinical Science* **78** (suppl. 2):92.

Thorogood, N (1990.) Caribbean home remedies and their importance for Black women's health care in Britain. In Abbott, P and Payne, G (eds) *New directions in the sociology of health*. London: Falmer.

Tilki, M (1994). Ethnic Irish older people. *British Journal of Nursing* **3**(17):909–13.

Treuherz, J, Cullinan, T R and Saunders, D I (1982). Determinants of infant-feeding practice in East London. *Human Nutrition: Applied Nutrition* **36A**:281–6.

Versi, E, Liu, K L, Chia, P and Seddon, G (1995). Obstetric outcome of Bangladeshi women in East London. *British Journal of Obstetrics and Gynaecology* **102**:630–7.

Viegas, O A C, Scott, P H, Cole, T J, Mansfield, H N, Wharton, P and Wharton, B A (1982a). Dietary protein energy supplementation of pregnant Asian mothers at Sorrento, Birmingham, I: Unselective during second and third trimesters. *British Medical Journal* **285**:589–92.

Viegas, O A C, Scott, P H, Cole, T J, Eton, P, Needham, P G and Wharton, B A (1982b). Dietary protein energy supplementation of pregnant Asian mothers at Sorrento, Birmingham, II: Selective during third trimester only. *British Medical Journal* **285**:592–5.

Wallace, B, Ahmed, R and Iqbal, S (1992). Nutrition and child development: a Healthy Communities Initiative with Bangladeshi and Pakistani women. *Community Health Action* **22**(10).

Ward, R J, Abraham, R, McFadyen, I R, Haines, A D, North, W R S, Patel, M and Bhatt, R V (1988). Assessment of trace metal intake and status in a Gujerati pregnant Asian population and their influence on the outcome of pregnancy. *British Journal of Obstetrics and Gynaecology* **95**:676–82.

Wardle, J, Wrightson, K and Gibson, L (1996). Body fat distribution in South Asian women and children. *International Journal of Obesity* **20**:267–71.

Warrington, S and Storey, D M (1988a). Comparative studies on Asian and Caucasian children, 1: Growth. *European Journal of Clinical Nutrition* **42**:61–7.

—— (1988b). Comparative studies on Asian and Caucasian children, 2: Nutrition, feeding practices and health. *European Journal of Clinical Nutrition* **42**:69–80.

Way, S (1991). Food for Asian mothers-to-be. *Nursing Times* **87**(49):50–2.

Wharton, P and Wharton, B (1989). Nutrition of Asian children: fetus and newborn. In Cruickshank, J K and Beevers, D G (eds.) *Ethnic factors in health and disease.* London: Wright, pp. 235–40.

Wharton, P A, Eaton, P M and Wharton, B (1984). Subethnic variation in the diets of Moslem, Sikh and Hindu pregnant women at Sorrento Maternity Hospital, Birmingham. *British Journal of Nutrition* **52**:469–76.

White, A, Freeth, S and O'Brien, M (1992). *Infant feeding 1990.* London: HMSO.

Williams, R G A (1992). The health of the Irish in Britain. In Ahmad, W (ed.) *The politics of race and health.* Bradford: Race Relations Research Unit.

Williams, R G A (1993a). Can data on Scottish Catholics tell us about descendants of the Irish in Scotland? A research note. *New Community* **19**:296–310.

Williams, R G A (1993b). The health costs of Britain's industrialization: a perspective from the Celtic periphery. In Platt, S, Thomas, H, Scott, S and Williams, G (eds) *Locating health: sociological and historical explorations.* Aldershot: Avebury, pp. 179–204.

Williams, R G A, Bhopal, R S and Hunt, K (1993). Health of a Punjabi ethnic minority in Glasgow: a comparison with the general population. *Journal of Epidemiology and Community Health* **47**:96–102.

Williams, R G A (1994). Britain's regional mortality: a legacy from disaster in the Celtic periphery? *Social Science and Medicine* **39**(2):189–99.

Williams, R G A, Bhopal, R S and Hunt, K. (1994). Coronary risk in a British Punjabi population: comparative profile of non-biochemical factors. *International Journal of Epidemiology* **23**(1):28–37.

Williams, S A, Sahota, P and Fairpo, C G (1989). Infant feeding practices within white and Asian communities in inner-city Leeds. *Journal of Human Nutrition and Dietetics* **2**:325–38.

Woollett, A, Dosanjh, N, Nicolson, P, Marshall, H, Djhanbakhch, O and Hadlow, J (1995). The ideas and experiences of pregnancy and childbirth of Asian and non-Asian women in East London. *British Journal of Medical Psychology* **68**:65–84.

Wright, M E (1995). A case-control study of maternal nutrition and neural tube defects in Northern Ireland. *Midwifery* **11**:146–52.